The

Real

Truth

Get**O**ver**D**arkness**G**et**O**ff**D**rugs**G**o**O**n**D**reaming
**Deliver Yourself From Darkness Into Your
Sunshine**

The

Real

Truth

Get**O**ver**D**arkness **G**et**O**ff**D**rugs **G**o**O**n**D**reaming

Deliver Yourself From Darkness Into Your Sunshine

DANA AXELROD

The Real Truth
By Dana Axelrod
Copyright © August 2022

ISBN:

Edited and formatted by Jenny Margotta:
editorjennymargotta@mail.com

Printed in United States of America

Dedication

To my "Priceless Blessings"

Ahlam, Jennifer, Jessie, Gracelyn, and Ella

Table of Contents

INTRODUCTION 1

Mac 3

Philosophy of Addiction 7

Recovery 15

FOUNDATIONAL TOOLS 30

Introduction to Foundational Tools 32

Believe 37

Faith 41

No Doubts 46

Mental Discipline..52

Relentless Commitment..58

Self-Motivation...66

Summary of Foundational Tools 71

CLASSES 74

Revolution..76

Words..91

Wants Versus Needs 105

Affirmations...111

Smart Versus Strong 135

Role Models..148

Choice 158

Q & A and Additional Thoughts...........................171

SPIRITUALITY 190

GetOffDrugs 192

Soulo and the Spirit Whisperer............................197

God's Buffet...205

God is the Silence Between Peaceful Thoughts 211

ABOUT THE AUTHOR 220

THANKS AND REMEMBRANCES............................223

INTRODUCTION

Mac

Mac: I was standing, looking out at the city lights from my condo. This city was beautiful at night.

I was thinking how I had reached this level of success in seven years. I should be proud, somewhat happy, and at peace with myself. I was once all these things. What had changed within me, I wondered?

My clientele, my business, and my family relationships had not suffered at all. If anything, all these things had improved.

The reality was that I was the one who was suffering internally.

My business clientele revolved around and consisted of customer satisfaction based on positive customer relationships. I had never been more in demand and respected by others. In addition, the raising of my fees had done little to slow down my calendar of appointments. I had accomplished everything I set out to do. Don't get me wrong, things did not come easy. My clients and profits were simply a summation of all the energy I had put into my goals.

Regrettably, I had lost my energy and focus, that "drive" to keep pushing myself daily. At that time, I was unable to find my way back to any type of goal or to motivate myself. There was a time in which I had readily accomplished every set of goals I had. My thought process for each step toward these goals never wavered. Now, I couldn't think of, see, or feel any desire to set new goals, and I wasn't really committed to the goals I had already achieved. To say I was less than satisfied with my efforts would be an understatement. I was starting to get really concerned about why I felt this way. It was if I found myself slipping away and heading to a free-fall straight down.

I was most certainly attuned to this situation. Nevertheless, I found myself a passenger on this spiraling ride, unwilling or uncertain how to take control of this predicament. I was fully aware that if I didn't find a way to change, I would end up again at the destination of nowhere.

At one time I was a hopeless alcoholic, compulsive gambler, and I abused any drug that came my way. I had lost everything: wife, kids, good job, and most importantly . . . I lost myself. In losing myself, I was simply another homeless addict surviving in the bleak, addictive world of chaos, despair, and dysfunction. I had become a resident of this dark metropolis without even being conscious and aware of how I managed to travel to this spot of existence in so little time. It was like one day I woke up under a pile of cardboard. I was sick, no money, and no clue as to what I had been doing the past years to get to this miserable destination.

I look back, amazed how someone like myself had accepted this dreary, ongoing outcome and allowed it to keep happening. At the time I did not realize or admit I was the cause of these circumstances.

I understand and realize, of course, that my problem was one of complacency and lack of effort. I had recently acknowledged to myself that my enthusiasm had waned, I lacked energy, and had no passion to continue at the pace I once set for myself. I was thinking I was too smart to relapse on substances, although my old, destructive thoughts and negative behaviors were starting to reappear.

The continuous red flags were sprouting up and I could not ignore them any longer. I began thinking back and asking myself how I had managed to get out of a life nearly destroyed and make it to where I was now standing. The simple answer hit me then. I felt a sudden bolt of lightning erupting inside the synopses of my brain. I could feel the hum of energy instantly "kick starting" my thoughts. I knew the

Real Truth. I knew The Answer to my problem. It was here, hovering at the edge of my consciousness all the time.

Even though I was in self-imposed, ego-driven denial, the answer had always been to re-engage with the man who showed me how to pick myself up and succeed after my near-death crash landing. Of course, I refer to my old counselor, teacher, mentor, Mr. Dana.

It had been years since I had contacted him. Perhaps it was embarrassment, guilt, or simply that I thought I did not need him any more in my life. Maybe my escalating success had prevented me from reaching out to him until now. Most likely, knowing Mr. Dana, he would say it was something along those lines, along with pride and ego.

For the moment, I was proud of myself. I could not remember the last time I could say I that. I had seen the warning signs. This time I decided to do something about this continuing malady which was becoming more prevalent in my life. I had felt deep inside myself the momentum changing and heading in the wrong direction. Without any doubt, this inevitable direction would lead to the pavement covered in cardboard. I needed a recalibration of my spirit, a refresher of what had helped me achieve my success. I needed a practicum in the Real Truth taught by Mr. Dana.

Reaching out to this man was easier than expected. After a tongue-tied fifteen minutes, I explained my issues, with full disclosure and transparency. The one thing I did know was that I must always be in the Real Truth when talking to Mr. Dana. This was especially true when it came to my escalating, negative thoughts and issues. In a matter of moments, I was overcome with excitement when I heard Mr. Dana's voice singing on the phone. I was now rearranging my calendar. I was immediately headed for deep, serious, re-education and rejuvenation. I was leaving now. Let this new journey begin!

0

The following essays, notes, classes, thoughts, and talks are a direct result of my observations stemming from Mr. Dana allowing me to question him about my new doubts and "shadow" him throughout his day.

In some cases a slight edit or combination of personal talks with classes have been made. The meaning, depth, and concepts have not been altered or changed. These direct observations were made over the course of an intensive two weeks and with the approval of anyone mentioned in the following pages.

Philosophy of Addiction

As I began to get further involved with Mr. Dana and his educational teachings on productive change, I was curious about his philosophy and his approach to the addict or anyone who was floundering or stagnant in their life and desiring motivation and positive change. I asked Mr. Dana if he could educate the clients on what he felt were the cornerstones of being an addict and what addiction was.

Mr. Dana started explaining his viewpoints to the class of clients by stressing he was a "philosopher of addiction." Also, he would illuminate positive change to the individual through practiced concepts, which included spirituality. These concepts, applied by any person eager to obtain a better life through committed, daily practice, will be successful and the person will see change within. Mr. Dana emphasized that *Recovery*, along with a better life, happens gradually and is a long-term process which must be continued "until."

Mr. Dana went on to explain how he used everything and anything to make his point. He also wanted me and the class to understand that he would elaborate on "the story" to fit his perspective. He said, "It is not really the story per se; it is the message from the story and my interpretation of the story to teach positive change and illustrate my points." Continuing, he clearly stated that he would use any subject he could to make his point on addiction in order to help the clients succeed and obtain the goal of being addiction free and obtain a better life.

He further elaborated by stating, "I will teach and

elevate your minds by using such subjects as history, art, sports, mythology, religion, spiritual teachings, world events, science, etc. And by using my personal interpretations and opinions, I will weave them together to create my own philosophy to instill knowledge and profound change in anyone." He went on to say, "These concepts are used to develop daily life skills, with the result being a quality of life in which you are able to find joy, peace, and balance. You need not be an addict; although directed primarily at addicts, these concepts and tools will allow any individual to enjoy life.

Without any hesitation, I jumped right in I asked his opinion. "What is addiction and how is someone defined as an addict?"

Mr. Dana responded in a normal, factual voice, addressing me along with the class. "I have found that addiction is based on two very simple criteria: tolerance and withdrawal." He then went on to explain the criteria.

The first criteria is tolerance of the addict. Does the addict, after being in the addiction, need more quantity to achieve the same effect? In other words, is the quantity continuing to go up and the addict needs more of that particular addiction to reach the same high or feeling? Is the quantity escalating and the addict only maintaining a status quo to simply function?

If the answer is not a resounding, "No," then you have met the first criteria.

The second criteria is based on the withdrawal phase. Do you have any physical symptoms of withdrawal? Do you have any emotional symptoms of withdrawal? Do you have any mental symptoms of withdrawal?

Clients asked him to expand a bit on each of the aforementioned, and Mr. Dana replied, "Let's pretend you are an addict of any type and go 'without your addiction' for a period of time, say twenty-four hours. More than likely, physically, you will experience symptoms of sweating, shakes, nausea, vomiting, sleeplessness or too much sleep, or loss of appetite. This is your addiction controlling you physically. Let's say you have no negative symptoms. Maybe you just have a need to go out and actively partake in your addiction by going to the casino, meeting your dealer, etc. This is another basic concept of control. When anything controls you, it is a loss of personal freedom. Your addiction is making you choose to become physically involved. To me this is the classic definition of control: not having freedom to do what you really desire."

Mr. Dana continued, quite seriously, "I will give you a real example of control. This is a true story. Now, I am only talking about myself, not any of you. I need to make this point extremely clear right off the bat. Again, I am not talking about any of you." He gestured to all the clients. "In my addiction, I was the biggest whore, bitch, chump, fool, trick, or punk. I would sit with my darling wife alone on a Friday night, with plans to be alone and get really romantic, as the kids were gone for the evening, which was a rarity. I truly desired to get close and intimate with this beautiful, sexy women. As I lit candles and put some early Sinatra on the stereo, I started telling my wife wonderful things. I told her about how nothing would ever come before her. I was enjoying this magical moment when all of a sudden, out of nowhere, a voice in my head would scream, 'Hey, you fucking bitch, get dressed right now and put your shoes on! You are not going to be sitting on the couch with your wife. Get the fuck up now, punk! You are going to go to work for me, your addiction, by going out for the night and into the street to score some dope.'

"I could not ignore this voice in my head, regardless of how hard I tried over and over not to listen to it. This voice

9

would be screaming so loudly in my mind that I was surprised my wife did not hear. The voice continued in my head, screaming, 'You fucking whore, get your bitch ass out on the street now! You are not staying home with your gorgeous wife. You're my slave and you will do what I am telling you to do. Move your ass now!'

"Looking around, I came to the eventual conclusion and realization that my addiction was my pimp in my head, controlling me and telling me what to do. I could never escape, as I was enslaved, and my addiction was the tyrannical master. I listened, obeyed, and did what I was ordered to do by my pimp every time. This did not happen once or twice—it happened all the time I was in my addiction. Again and again, over and over, throughout the years of my addiction, I simply obeyed without hesitation. This is due to the fact that I was a beaten-down slave who had given up all hope of any chance to escape.

"Not only was I tremendously disappointing my wife and family, the real casualty was myself and my future. The feelings of shame, guilt, and profound emptiness in that failure were deeply etched and embedded in my spirit and psyche, the result being the darkest, deepest disappointment that I locked inside myself.

"This slavery was self-imposed and self-inflected. The only way to rid myself of this haunting, personal doom was to engage and immerse myself even more fully in my addiction. Talk about a never-ending, vicious cycle! The worst part was that I was fully aware of this, and due to my personal embarrassment, I could not and would not ask anyone for help. I instinctually pretended on the outside to anyone and everyone that everything was 'okay' and I was 'alright.' But on the inside, I was consumed by these negative, self-inflicted feelings of despair. I was always so alone with these thoughts and feelings and believed there with no way out except for death.

"During all the years in my addiction, I am lucky to only have one regret in my life. I have been married for thirty-eight years and have been clean and in recovery for the last twelve of those thirty-eight years. These twelve years in recovery have been like a honeymoon for me. I am truly blissful and so extremely blessed to have such a fantastic, supportive, giving, loving wife. I am so grateful for her every single day. I could have had this women every single day for thirty-eight years. I blew the first twenty-five years of my marriage due to my addiction. How fucked up is that? That is my one and only regret!"

Continuing in a deep, remorseful tone, Mr. Dana said, "On other occasions I would wake up, stumble out of bed, and see my children dressed in their Disneyland shirts and Mickey Mouse hats.

"In unison my children would excitedly scream, 'We're ready! Daddy. you said last night to get ready early, as we're all going to Disneyland.'

"Now, I would have every intention of fulfilling this promise at the moment, but as I was about to get ready, a loud, knocking voice in my head would say, "Bitch, you ain't going to Disneyland. You need to go out on the street and score some dope or you going to be sick." Again, it was my pimp ordering me to lie once again to my children and pursue my addiction. The worst part in all of this was that my children stopped trusting me and believing me, and it took a very long time to regain their trust."

In a sorrowful, mesmerizing voice, he continued, " I *always* listened and obeyed without resistance to my addiction, this pimp in my head! Now, I am only saying that *I* was these terrible things. You all have to be *really truthful* with yourselves and tell yourselves honestly what you were in your addictions. You need to do this regardless of the pain, guilt, shame, or embarrassment caused by confronting the truth about yourself. Be real and concentrate on how badly you want to change this negative label you put on yourselves. Listen, and hear this really well, all of you, and remember this and know this, as I want to make this last and important point very, very clear. *I am no one's bitch or whore today. I am free!*"

Mr. Dana proceeded to state, "The addict actively choses to 'seek' when choosing addiction over responsibilities or positive options, refusing to choose wonderful blessings like family time, work, dinner, or any productive engagement first. The addict *always* choses the addiction first. *Always*, regardless of the consequences.

"Simply put, the addict who chooses to go and seek the addiction is being "physically" controlled. The addict has lost all personal freedoms.

"Then again, perhaps the addict does not have any of these aforementioned physical symptoms. That's fine. The addict has no 'physical withdrawals.'

"However, say the addict does have irritability, anxiety, confusion, depression, or mood swings. That would meet the criteria of emotional withdrawal. Remember, any type or form of withdrawal—physical, emotional, or mental—meets the criteria.

"Perhaps the addict has no physical withdrawal and no emotional withdrawal. The addict chooses to go to work; the addict is quite calm and exhibits stable emotions. Is the addict mentally consumed? Does the addict think all day about going to his addiction? Does the addict think about how he is going to get his addiction satisfied? Does the addict make plans about the addiction? The bottom line is this: Does the addict allow thoughts of addiction to consume the mind all day instead of concentrating on the task at hand and or being present and in the moment? That is mental addiction.

"That is what addiction is, and addiction's mission is to devour your spirit from within, with the result of any addiction being spiritual erosion, emotional homicide, and the amputation of dreams. The totality of addiction is having a life of deep pain, regretful misery, and most importantly, a loss of freedom.

"Addicts need to understand and know the human spirit was not made to be cowardly trapped and locked in a self-imposed cage deep within oneself. In the addiction, the spirit is beaten down daily, drugged non-stop. The spirit is bordering on extinction and oblivion while remaining unconscious. The spirit is a silent witness to one's internal demise. The addict is woefully aware of this and does nothing to prevent the unthinkable from happening. The addict is quite in touch with this fact and continues on the path of a walking, living suicide.

"No addicts are proud of themselves and where they have ended up. Addicts do not grow up wanting to be a disappointment to themselves and others around them. Nevertheless, addicts find themselves in a wasted graveyard of broken dreams with their spirits shattered.

"Every addict is unwilling to confront himself/herself by accepting the responsibility of how he/she has ended up alone in the middle of nowhere.

"Growing up, every addict had dreams, an imagination. All of us played with sticks and dirt and made it exciting. Growing up, there was electricity in the air, and everything, everywhere, seemed so magical. The spirit is supposed to be able to soar untethered, to fly, knowing and walking in truth. The spirit is the moral compass within, telling oneself to always do the right thing and pursue greatness and follow one's dreams. We live through our consciousness. The addiction renders one's spirit unconscious.

"Recovery reactivates one's dreams and imagination. In recovery, one can go back to being a dreamer and take actions to begin to live and follow the path to their dreams again. Our spirit knows what to do. Recovery allows the spirit to wander the Earth.

"The key is to simply start. Just begin, as beginning *is* a new start forward and, finally, in the right direction."

Mr. Dana ended the session by saying, "To quote Lao Szu, the journey of a thousand miles begins with the first step." Mr. Dana gave a heartfelt thanks to everyone for listening and walked out with applause following him.

Recovery

Mac: It was almost a "new" house at the facility. I wanted to see the effects of Mr. Dana's classes on the new clients. As usual, there were several of the staff sitting at the back wall. A few were Mr. Dana's past clients who now were counselors. To my surprise, I noticed the administrator for all the Southern California facilities sitting unobtrusively in the back. Hmmm.

I remember wondering, "Why is she here?"

0

Mr. Dana began. "Good morning, all you beautiful people. Today, I want to first talk to all of you about what the word recovery means. I do not mean recovery with regard to addiction. Rather, what does the word recovery mean outside of addiction and in everyday life?"

Mr. Dana went to the blackboard and preceded to write the word RECOVER in big, bold, black letters. Underneath the word RECOVER he then wrote:

1) Regaining what was lost or stolen.

Then he wrote:

2) Finding that which is missing.

And finally, he wrote:

3) To Restore to new or original.

Continuing his lecture, he then simply gave examples of each by saying, "I am going to *recover* the 'black box' from the Malaysian airliner that went missing in

15

the Indian Ocean.

"I am going to *recover* Magellan's gold treasure that sank in the year 1510.

"I am going to *recover* and restore the upholstery on this 1955 Cadillac convertible.

"You see, all of you have this chance in recovery to regain what you lost by finding inside yourself what has been lost, missing, and definitely stolen by your addition. In recovery you begin to restore yourself to your natural state of being by becoming the person you were once destined to be. With continued practice, you will *recover* what your addiction stole from you in one form or another. Unfortunately, you will never ever recover life's most precious gift, which is your time. Your addiction has stolen the most valuable gift God has granted you . . . time. Be honest and real about all the time you personally wasted in your addiction.

"Speaking for myself, I spent over thirty hard-core years in my addiction as an alcoholic, drug addict, and degenerate gambler, and I realize I do not know how much time I have left in this life. I absolutely refuse to waste any more of my time now. Today, I am extremely judicial when it comes to expending my time on anything insignificant or meaningless. I won't get any of my time back, ever, so I use this new knowledge as an advantage by avoiding senseless drama, arguments, gossip, and petty events that unfold daily in any person's life, including my own. The last thing I want to do is waste this priceless, extremely limited commodity on the pointless pursuit of nothing that will not really matter or count in the overall scheme of my life. I refuse, at the end of my life, to *wish* I had more time and *wish* I had done things differently in irrelevant situations which had no bearing on my life. I do not want to say, 'Where did the time go?' I now know this, and by knowing this, I practice daily to not react or respond to anything which does not have or will not have an overall positive effect on my future.

"It is so important to understand this point. We must all realize that none of us ever know how much actual time we have to live. Today, I refuse to waste one nanosecond of my time on trivial bullshit. On issues that are non-productive. I continue to practice how not to deal with them and keep practicing to not involve myself by avoiding these things that deplete my time on Earth. The result of this 'time practice' is that my life is getting free of frustration, resentments, anger, endless drama, gossip, and all the other negative distractions that devour my time and will detour me from achieving my goals quicker, along with the pursuit of my dreams. This judicial 'time practice' allows me to be more free with my mind and spirit, creating inner calm and peace. I have recovered more freedom and independence from outside negative forces by using my time wisely.

"As an ex-addict, everything except the gift of time is replaceable. Ex-addicts will recover and go on and get a new job or career, reconnect with their spouse or, eventually, get a new spouse. Lost your home or apartment? In recovery, the ex-addict will get a new dwelling. Over your lifelong, never-ending journey of recovery, the ex-addict will eventually regain their children. However, it will take a lot of hard work on your part for your child to start to trust you again. That is okay as well, as you, the ex-addict, has the rest of your life to regain this lost trust that was stolen by your addiction and to re-bond with your children. Ask yourselves, 'What did I lose? What is missing in my life? What do I want to regain?' Most importantly, ask yourself, 'What was stolen from me besides my time on Earth?' These are hard questions and when you have the answers, go out into this new life of *recovery* to regain the things that slipped away or were stolen from you by your addiction.

"Remember, in your addiction, almost everything 'fell out of place' and every addict knows why.

"By being honest, all addicts know 'the why.' Every addict knows why they went to jail, lost their job, lost their children to CFS, lost their spouse, their car, their health, etc., etc. If you are still in denial and continue to make excuses as to why these negative events always surrounded and occurred in your addiction, then you are not being real and will not succeed in recovery.

"Keep in mind that every AA and NA chip has inscribed on it, 'To Thy Own Self Be True.' In other words, stop lying to yourself. Recovery is about telling yourself the truth. I don't expect any of you to tell me the absolute truth. Why would you? However, if you really are ready for recovery, you must tell *yourself* the truth.

"Now is the time for honest self-assessment by being *really truthful* to self. You will always come up with the truthful answer by being extremely open and honest with yourself. If you are certain you desire change, are willing to put in effort, and want to end your addiction once and for all, now is the time for direct confrontation of self. No more bull shitting, no more denials. Stop the excuses. All that is required is simply flat, honest truth and full disclosure to yourself. You have always known the answer. As the renowned poet Sonya Kassam wrote, 'I create the poison and I am the cure.'

"Some of you lost your children, your spouse, your job, your house, your passion, your dreams, your personal freedom, and the most important thing . . . you lost *yourself*, along with your pure spirit. In your addiction you were unable to choose what was best for you. Addiction *decides* to choose what is the worst for you. Every choice we make in our addiction takes us further from the natural abundance of blessings that God provides. Our addiction leads us to penalties and consequences in which we lose these priceless blessings. You, the addict, if you are being honest, know why. We are doing the wrong things and going against natural harmony.

"In recovery, we do the right things, and these blessings which are priceless in value are always being attracted into our lives. Eventually, the ex-addict never asks the *why*. The ex-addict in recovery now knows the why. Remember, recovery means regaining, and you will eventually regain these things you now truly desire and lost or had stolen from you. As you slowly practice and begin acquiring and restoring these lost blessings into your life, it is important to know the reason why as well. The *why* is due to the fact that you are working hard and practicing doing the right thing! In recovery, things fall *into* place, not out of place. This is important to know. *Everything falls into place*, and now, by doing the right things instead of the wrong things, you are getting what you deserve. You are now moving with God's natural harmony."

Mr. Dana paused then asked the class, "How much is your life worth?"

Various clients in class shouted, "Priceless." "Worth everything." "Not enough money to buy me."

Mr. Dana asked the class in a straightforward tone, "How much are your children worth?"

Again, the class shouted, "Priceless."

Mr. Dana then called on Rico. "Rico, I see you have your hand up. Do you want to comment further?"

Rico was an extremely intimidating, thirty-two-year-old Hispanic male with teardrop tattoos coming out of the corner of each eye, along with 'ink' running down each arm. In a tough tone of voice, Rico said, "Nothing is worth more than my children. They mean everything to me. My children are priceless, like you say. I would take a bullet for them."

Mr. Dana looked at Rico and asked, "May I discuss you and your addiction in front of the class and ask you some *really truthful* questions?"

Rico nodded his head and, with a laugh, said, "Fire away, I got nothing to hide."

Mr. Dana walked slowly from the podium to the middle of the room and started a quiet chant, "Priceless, priceless, priceless. Priceless, you say? What was your drug of choice?"

Rico boastfully stated, "Meth, a lot of meth."

Continuing the questions in a very respectful manner, Mr. Dana then asked, "You ever get ripped off?"

In a hard voice and an even harder stare, Rico spit out, "Fuck no."

The entire class laughed, as they all knew Rico was considered someone not to mess with or play around with.

"You ever go to jail and do any time?"

Rico laughed and stated coldly and quickly, "Last time was two years . . . state, not county."

"How old are your girls, man?" Mr. Dana asked.

Rico: "Two daughters, eleven and nine."

Mr. Dana: "What was the last charge?"

Rico: "Violation of parole due to possession of meth."

Mr. Dana: "How much in dollar amount of meth?"

Rico: "Shit, man, it was only forty dollars or so."

Mr. Dana: "Your daughters went without a father for two years while you were locked up?"

Rico: "Yep."

Mr. Dana: "Where are the kids?"

Rico, looking sheepish and starting to frown, said quietly, "Don't know. My ex-wife took 'em and split while I was doing my last bit."

0

Mac: Mr. Dana began using his left hand as a scale by demonstrating the scale going lower and lower while chanting the word priceless over and over.

0

Mr. Dana: "Priceless, priceless, priceless."

0

Mac: Every time Mr. Dana said the word 'priceless,' his left hand would drop lower, pretending how much weight the word 'priceless' meant. And the right hand would go way down as the left hand went go up.

0

Mr. Dana: "Two years without your daughters." (Left hand going up and up.)

Then he said, "Priceless, priceless, priceless." (Right hand going way down to the ground.)

Mr. Dana: "Two years and forty dollars of meth." (He demonstrated with the left hand now over his head.)

Mr. Dana repeated, "Two years and forty dollars." Then he continued, "Rico, I know you well. We talk every day. I know you're a really tough, street-smart dude. Does this"—he gestured with both his hands—"make sense to you? You gave up two years of freedom, your purest asset— time—and your priceless children"—Mr. Dana emphasized 'priceless' with a look of puzzled bewilderment on his face— "for forty dollars?" In a warm, non-confrontational voice, he continued, "I thought you said 'fuck no' when I asked if you've been ripped off. Looks to me like your addiction ripped you the fuck off!"

21

The class laughed and clapped a bit as Rico looked a little embarrassed.

Speaking to the entire class, Mr. Dana said, "I don't know why most of you are laughing and clapping. You've all been fuckin' ripped off . . . worse than Rico and for less. At least Rico had the courage to be the only one to raise his hand and honestly tell the truth in front of all of you." Mr. Dana looked directly at Rico as he said, "Recovery requires courage. I have only respect for this man for demonstrating his willingness to be open and truthful."

Walking back to the podium, Mr. Dana continued, "All of you have to realize that, as addicts, we are always reinventing ourselves, changing ourselves like human chameleons. Every day, the addict plays the role of an actor by pretending that everything is okay and everything is fine. The addict always knows, deep in the soul, what the *real truth* really is. And that truth is, 'I am not okay and I have never known what being fine feels like.' If you think you are fine in your addiction, you need to rid yourself of that delusion and deniability and get *real* with yourself. That is the real reason addicts crave chaos and daily drama, as they know how to operate on that stage of drama and are always in control of the chaos.

"The addict, every day, all day, plays the role of a movie star. With the same exact lines from their movie script. The script of their autobiographical movie never changes. These lines are familiar and instinctually embedded in this counterfeit self. The addict has memorized his lines of lies perfectly and is always ready for improvisation, depending on the 'scene.' The movie rarely changes. Same scenes, same dialogue, same locations. The addict is like a fine jazz musician who has been soloing on the saxophone forever. The improvisation sounds fantastic after years practicing the same tune!

"The addict is always starring in the same role of always lying, living in chaos, getting into arguments, causing drama, and living in familiar dysfunction while basking in the personal spotlight of shame. The shame of losing their children"—nodding to Rico—"shame of losing their spouse, shame of losing their job. The biggest shame is losing their precious time. The shame of it all cumulates and causes the addict to harbor deep inside themselves the feeling that they are worthless and unworthy of deserving anything. Yet they addict always says, 'I am fine and okay.'"

Then Mr. Dana grabbed a blank sheet of paper, gesturing with it and reading in an "announcer's" voice: "And this year's Oscar again goes to . . . the addict, for his starring role in *My Tragic Life*." Then, in a hushed voice, he continued, "Accepting this year's Oscar for Best Starring Role is the addict's family, as the addict could not be here tonight because . . . the addict is dead. Talk about a realistic Academy performance! The addict won last year, as well, and could not attend then either as the addict was in jail."

Mr. Dana changed his voice and pretended to be the father of the addict. In a very solemn, mournful voice, he said, "At least my son, the addict, is now at peace . . . finally."

Mr. Dana proceeded to throw the papers in his hand into the air and shout, "At peace! At peace! I don't want to be at peace when I am fucking dead. Are you kidding me? That is what is said at every addict's funeral. 'At least they are at peace now.' I *want* peace right fucking *now*! When I am above the ground, not when I'm dead!"

He stopped and looked at everyone in the room. "If you listen to me and practice these things all the time, you will learn to be at peace *now*!"

0

Mac: Mr. Dana was now on a passionate roll. I knew from prior experience that nothing would get in his way.

0

Mr. Dana: "The addict is incapable of thinking, talking, or going in a straight, linear direction from point A to point B. Going from A to B is impossible for the addict. The addict is always going from point A to point G, then from G to point Y, then from Y to B. The addict is incapable of ever going in a straight line. The addict is always, always talking and saying absolutely nothing of value, while moving in circles. The addict is always in a hurry, always rushing, and never, ever, ever gets anywhere. Always cooking and nothing is ever in the pot. Anyone hearing this who thinks what I'm saying is bullshit, who denies what I'm saying, is still lost, missing, and close-minded. More importantly, they are continuing to fail again. The addict fails at failing, not even considering any other options or trying something different or new. Why? Due to the fact that it is not in the addict's fucking script, that's why.

"Recovery is a new foreign language in a new foreign country. This new land, with its customs and traditions, is only heard and talked about in hushed ridicule among other addicts. What does the addict say to those who have left the island of the walking dead of addiction and have made it to this healthy, living, foreign country and are now journeying in this new land? Addicts look at those who have succeeded and escaped addiction successfully and wish those successful travelers to have bad luck and an even worse fate after coming back from a life-changing destination. Can you imagine going on a lifelong vacation to a new foreign country called the Promised Land of the Recovered Living and someone tells you, 'I hope your airplane crashes with you and all your family on board and you all die?'

"The addict always says to this new, clean traveler, 'Hey, man, I got some really good shit. C'mon, let's get fucked up and wasted (so you can continue with me to ruin your life). I have known you a long time, you ain't gonna stay clean.' And so it goes. The addict always tries to talk someone out of beginning recovery.

"Why is this? It is due to the fact that the addict is threatened by someone who is willing to put in effort to change, someone who wants something new and better. The addict is frightened of someone leaving the ranks of addiction and entering a new unknown to learn and practice new thoughts and a new course of action by finally coming to a realization that they are worth more and are no longer willing to get ripped off by their addiction. "Ain't that right, Rico? Isn't that why you're all here? You're tired of getting ripped off, as it does not add up, and your addiction is profiting off your hopes and dreams.

"The addict is always so scared of anything new and unfamiliar beyond and outside of their control . . . with the real reason being . . . it's not in the script, and the addict has now lost another costar. The addict knows, deep down, that they are even further along and this is frightening.

"The addict desiring recovery should not be scared or threatened by these new customs, new traditions, new language in the country of Recovery. The recovering addict needs to learn they are misdiagnosing their feelings. They are mistaking being excited for being scared.

"How many of you or people you know would be scared or frightened to go on vacation and fly First Class to the Bahamas for free?" (He gestured to the class.)

"Recovery is a one-way First-Class ticket out of Hell. I love First Class, and some of you are putting in so little commitment and effort that you might be lucky to be put in the baggage compartment."

The class started whooping amid much laughter.

"As addicts, we speak and live on the island called Addiction. Addicts all know this language of addiction, they know the customs, the traditions. For instance, the custom of getting to the bar before two a.m. if you want a drink. The custom and tradition of don't ever bring a stranger to the dealer's house. Don't call my house after ten p.m. or talk in front of my spouse. It is common practice on the island of Addiction to say, 'Don't park in the driveway, don't hold the pipe over the dope because you will burn it,' as they teach the customer to spin the pipe.'

The class burst out in laughter.

"We follow these addictive traditions without ever questioning these customs. Why? If we want to survive on Addiction Island, we need to learn these things.

"Look, in my addiction, after continued practice and constant repetition, as time went by I got better at everything on the lonely island of Addiction. Practice, practice, practice. None of you started out as professional dope fiends or drunks. You practiced it. You got better at it. Remember when you got ripped off? Remember when you drove home drunk? Remember when you got shorted on the dope? Remember when you fronted the money to a friend, and you never saw that friend ever again? Now you hustlers are getting money fronted to you. *You* are doing the ripping off. *You* are shorting someone on the count. Why? You got better at it through practice, practice, practice. You learned the customs of addiction. Unfortunately, it was the wrong thing to practice and to learn. But ain't we good at it now?"

The entire class laughed.

Continuing, Mr. Dana said, "We became the principle inhabitants and elected ourselves rulers of this dark, distant land. Isolated on the island of Addiction, we moved right in, and after mastering this culture through ongoing, everyday practice, we started changing some traditions and customs of Addiction Island. All of you, make no mistake, it *is* a lonely island, quite far and away from civilization."

Mr. Dana then said he would speak the language of addicts. He began slowly, saying, "After crashing, called OG for some shit. Went to OG's crib, OG and I chopped it up, scored two doves, got my rig and tripped out.

"We all know—he pointed to the class—"what I just said, but I will interpret for those who don't speak this foreign language. 'I woke up, called my dealer for some drugs, went to his house, talked for a while, spent forty dollars to get my drugs, used my syringe, and got high as a motherfucker.'"

The class was now hooting and laughing

"See, you all speak and understand the foreign language of addiction," Mr. Dana said.

In an inquiring voice, he asked, "How many of you have ever been to another country? Hmmm . . . not many, I see. I'll tell you a true story. When I went to the Middle East for the first time, I did not speak one word of Arabic. I didn't panic; I wasn't scared. I was excited. There was magic in the air. I remember running up to everyone, asking questions and understanding absolutely nothing. I would point and pantomime to make myself understood. After a period of time, something strange happened. I could put a few pigeon sentences together. Eventually, after much trial and error, slowly, very slowly, I began to ask very basic questions. Some of these questions were, Where's the bathroom? How much is this? How do I get a taxi? How do I get to the beach? I could speak English all I wanted and no one understood it. I had to change and learn how to speak Arabic, all day, every

27

day. I learned the customs, the traditions of the Arabic world."

0

Mac: Suddenly, Mr. Dana began speaking Arabic fluently, to the surprise of all the clients and myself.

0

Mr. Dana asked, "Anyone know what I just said? Of course not. Why? You never needed to know Arabic. It is a foreign language. The same goes for recovery. Learn the language of recovery. Learn the traditions, the culture, and the customs. Remember, recovery is about open mindedness and accepting new concepts and knowledge. It *is* foreign to the addict. This is a new foreign language with words, customs, and traditions that we don't understand yet as addicts who desire recovery. All this foreign talk about spirit, truth, journey, honesty, integrity, dreams, hope. What is hope? Hope is simply the expectation that things will be better. Recovery brings you these new foreign concepts. Recovery implements these concepts into your life and character, making your life run smoother rather than rougher.

"The *harder* choice is almost always the right choice. The Land of Recovery is a very hard choice, and not doing anything about your addiction is extremely easy. All of you must practice this new way daily by being fully committed each and every day, all day, in order to achieve full recovery.

All of you have dreamed of this moment, and now the moment is here. Some of you, through your words and actions, demonstrate you are not ready for this 'defining moment' to better your life. This defining moment is this one moment which changes your character for the better.

Everyone wants better. Better transportation, better shoes, something better to eat, better dope—"

The class burst out laughing again. When the laughter died down, Mr. Dana resumed talking. "In recovery, we all get better at coping with everyday life, and our lives get better. For the addict, getting by and surviving is a way of life. For those in recovery, it's not about getting by and surviving, it's about being alive, striving, and thriving.

"Being alive, striving, thriving . . . a foreign language. Learn how to live in the Land of Recovery by practicing all day, every day, and you won't end up being a momentary tourist—you will be a native of this land."

And with that, Mr. Dana simply said, "Thank you for allowing me to talk to you. Class over."

Ongoing cheers followed Mr. Dana as walked out of the classroom.

0

Mac: I was lightheaded, dizzy with excitement. I knew I was on my way to revitalizing myself again. I took out my personal notebook and starting writing new thoughts and applications for work. It had been a very long time since I'd had these creative thoughts, let alone written them down.

FOUNDATIONAL TOOLS

Introduction to Foundational Tools

Mac: I was early. I noticed a few of the clients running to the empty seats in the first few rows. Mr. Dana always preached change. He always said, "If you want to really change and learn, you need to stop sitting in the back of the class. Sit up front, where you can absorb without distraction." Almost all the new clients were "stretched out" in the back rows.

0

Mr. Dana began speaking. "Good morning, class. Most of you are on the first cycle of this ninety-day in-house program. For those of you who have either been in this program before or have heard these classes previously, that's a good thing. Repetition is a great thing. Some of you might ask why. Repetition creates patterns. If all of you listen to these classes and use the foundational tools repeatedly, they will change your old patterns. I will continue to reference the salient points by interchanging certain themes in the next few classes. Repeating myself *is* intentional. All of you must realize that in your addiction you repeated your thoughts and actions all the time. What you really created were negative patterns.

"I will show you to use these foundational tools in a positive way to rid yourselves of these negative patterns and develop new ones. The principles are developmental in character. Developmental is the process of something being developed. I look at the word in another way."

0

Mac: Mr. Dana went to the blackboard and wrote the word

32

"Development." Then he inserted the word "Mental" in front of it."

0

Mr. Dana continued. "That's right. The words are 'mental development.' You need to develop these foundational tools with your mind. All of you must be present and totally aware of your thoughts at all times and implement these tools daily here in the program. Don't wait for tomorrow or make excuses. You need to do it right now . . . today.

"It is amazing to me how most of you wished for another chance to get your life on track during your addiction. I'm going to tell you something—your wish has come true. But a lot of you now are saying to yourself, 'I'm not ready. I didn't mean *now*' or some insane, crazy shit like that. Take advantage of this situation. You're here anyway. Your wish has been granted by God.

"I'm going to make all of you a bet."

0

Mac: Mr. Dana took his lanyard with his residential ID on it and held it up for all of the class to see.

0

In a serious tone, Mr. Dana said, "I will bet my entire reputation of being counselor of the year—twice—with the award of healer of the year, along with my ID, to any of you who practices these foundational tools for the ninety days you are in the program and thirty days after the program. If these foundational tools do not work, you can have my ID.

"Really, I ain't bullshitting you. I have been making this bet for over ten years here. All of you will notice that I

33

still have my original ID. I'm gonna tell you why. Those who didn't practice these tools in the program and after they left the program are now sitting in this class again, back in their full-blown addiction, miserable. And some are dead. Those who practiced these tools are now in recovery, living the life God guaranteed them. A lot of them have become counselors, and you may know them.

"Look, all of you are going to get recovery. Every single one of you ... or you will be dead. There is no middle ground.

"Now, I know addicts who are not dead and they are in their sixties. The problem is that they get up five times a night to piss. They shit in their pants, they go to the doctor every week and have failing health. Is that really living? Addiction is a slow suicide to the grave. It is *death on the installment plan.*

"The question is do you want recovery now or in ten years? The question I present to all of you is this: How do you think the ten years in between are going to be? Honestly, think about it, and tell yourself how much worse your life will be. It is certainly not going to be better. It is called 'quality of life.' How do you think the quality of life or the *in between* will be? C'mon, be honest. Anyone who thinks and says it will be better is full of shit.

"You see, your entire future is at stake. You *can* change your future. Let me ask you all a question. If you hadn't come into the program, what would your future hold for you as an addict?" Mr. Dana pointed to Alfredo.

"Ahh, to be really honest, in jail," Alfredo responded. "Or dead, probably dead. I'm lucky to be here right now."

When Mr. Dana pointed to Bianca, her answer was, "I would be dead. Like my husband or my mom. Dead, no doubt about it."

"Emilio?" Mr. Dana asked.

"I've already OD'd twice," Emilio said. "I know I should already be dead."

Mr. Dana continued, "Thank you for being honest. You see, you all know how to predict your future. Every addict knows the *real truth* about their future and where they were heading. To the grave. Dead. Graveyards are filled with the wasted hopes and dreams of addicts. The foundational tools in this program will help you change your future and lead you in a new direction.

"Your future is in your hands now. Take hold of it and change it. Remember what Mohammad says in the Koran: 'The mountain is not coming to me, I must go to the mountain.' Your future is *not* coming to you. You must go to it! The only way to change the future of an addict is through positive change and by grasping these new concepts.

"All of you who deep down want recovery must *think* about what I am saying at all times and implement these concepts immediately into your life.

"THINK is an acronym, and here's what it means. Mr. Dana went to the blackboard and wrote the following:

To Have Intellectual New Knowledge

Mr. Dana then said, "You all must memorize what THINK stands for. There will be a test at the end of the week. Anyone who passes the test gets extra phone time on Saturday. Also, you need to know what THUNK means as well." He went back to the blackboard and wrote:

To Have Unused New Knowledge

Mr. Dana continued in a forceful manner, "These tools are like muscles. Starting tomorrow, I will give you *new knowledge* by going into depth on each of the six foundational tools.

"Ok, that's it for today. Don't rush out immediately to go smoke or play ping pong. Take a moment to *think* about what you absorbed today.

"Or go run and smoke and *thunk* about it. Your choice. I did my job today, which is to educate all of you on positive change." As Mr. Dana began to walk out the side door, he simply said, "Class over."

Believe

"The war is won before it is fought."

—Lau Tsu

Mac: I was up all night, working on my accounts with a new sense of purpose. I didn't question why I had a sudden urge to touch base with my clientele. I knew why. Of course it was due to the new stimuli being offered in Mr. Dana's classes. I was the living proof of his teachings. Any client desiring in their heart change only needed to listen intently and apply what they learned."

0

Mr. Dana: "First, in order to understand, we all must agree upon a definition of the word 'believe.' To believe in oneself is to be able to count on oneself. Rely on oneself and trust in one's abilities by having confidence in one's choices. The importance of believing in oneself cannot be understated. It is one of the main components or building blocks of the foundational tools of recovery.

"This is never easy for the addict, as it takes practice to recognize even the slightest steps forward and obtaining positive results. This is due to the simple fact that an addict is always undermining themselves by lacking a true belief in what they are doing, regardless of whether their actions are of a positive nature or a negative one. Now add into this equation the countless others who once relied on you and have stopped believing in you as well. The addict's family, friends, peers, employers, co-workers, etc. arrived at this conclusion based on all the addict's negative actions in the pursuit of their addictions. The addict's façade of everything is 'fine and okay' has been pierced by the truth based on their own negative actions. Everyone they were close to has stopped being able to rely on them. This contributes to a total lack of trust in the addict's own actions and motives when undertaking any type of task, and it is especially true in the addiction.

"It is impossible for an addict to trust and believe in themselves, as the addict is always conscious of the lying, cheating, and deceiving of their own spirit with those close to and associating with the addict.

"The addict's lack of self-belief rocks him and penetrates the core of what is remaining of a once wholesome, God-giving foundation of spirit based on instinctual right and wrong. This is also evident when the addict is on the way to participating in events related to their addiction or actually participating in their addiction.

"Addicts are always questioning the circumstances they find themselves in. The addict on longer seems to have a firm conviction in any of their abilities. This includes the seeking out and the procurement of their addiction. The addict is constantly questioning self and wondering if the addictive journey will actually take place. All day, every day, a relentless assault on the mind and soul takes place, further shattering into pieces this God-given foundation.

"This onslaught culminates in the endless, internal questioning of the outcome of their addictive journey, the bizarre result being a lack of belief in the results of addiction *while they are in it*!

"Therefore, as an addict, it is very difficult to truly rely on one's own crippled, decision-making capabilities. The constant daily bombardment of negative thoughts increases the addict's personal insecurities, which are linked with a decline of moral values. The addict's mind and diseased spirit before, during , and after the initial contact of their addiction continue to face an internal barrage of negativity. This negativity is accompanied by a strong force of disguised, mental unease which makes it impossible to trust and believe in oneself. At all times, this negative, chaotic thinking storms away in one's psyche and continues to crash against any remaining remnants of positivity of character and moral fiber. The end result is the daily, ongoing, internal corrosion of emotional coping mechanisms, an erosion of a positive belief system, elimination of instinctual choices, and an eclipsing of what was once a receptive spirit.

"In recovery, when the journey is in its initial phase, the addict must simply recognize and maintain a desire within self to change for the better. At first the addict only has to slightly begin to believe that change is possible. *Begin to believe.* The *first* step. Taking this one step is the spark of energy that creates positive momentum.

"The addict in recovery must be aware of a strong, negative resistance from within and counter this force by remembering the reasons why they have finally sought out recovery. In recovery, the battle within one's entire being rages persistently. The addict must understand that by choosing recovery, in all actuality they are finally, after years of denial, relenting and admitting to themself the *real truth.* This real truth is the recognition of self-inflicted pain and the horrors that their addiction has caused in life. The addict is finally admitting truthfully to self what they have always known personally about their addiction. Their addiction is *death on the installment plan.*

"The addict must begin to believe that positive change will happen within them. The addict must begin to believe they are capable of obtaining their personal freedoms again by relinquishing their addiction. This is the start to the overall success of recovery. A simple belief is all that is required to throw off the shackles of addiction.

"Remember, simple does not mean easy. Without a belief that they are capable of exterminating their old addictive system of thought, habits, and actions, recovery cannot and will not be obtained. It is time for the addict to stop covering up for the addiction. It is time for the addict to believe and stand up for recovery.

"Class is now over."

0

Mac: with that, Mr. Dana simply walked out of class.

Faith

Mac: Mr. Dana walked into the class. At the podium he faced all the clients in the class and made an exaggerated prayer by putting both hands to his lips and kissing his hands. Then he raised his hands over his head and looked up.

0

Mr. Dana yelled, "THANK YOU, GOD!"

0

Mac: The clients immediately sat up straight in their chairs and paid rapt attention. I have noticed that, unlike in other facilitator's classes, the clients in Mr. Dana's classes don't cross-talk or get up to leave for the bathroom. It seems that Mr. Dana gives the clients respect and has earned the clients' respect as well. I imagine it is due to Mr. Dana always being truthful, genuine, and always available to clients, regardless of what he has going on. Mr. Dana has repeatedly stated, "Unless I am with another client, nothing is more important than you. I will never tell you to come back or that I am busy. This is a promise."
Also, the one class I attended where a client was talking, Mr. Dana shut him down so quickly that it has not happened again, at least not that I have noticed. In this residential facility, word travels faster than a heartbeat to new clients and that word is: "Don't fuck around in Mr. Dana's classes or with Mr. Dana unless you want a problem with all of us."
It appears that Mr. Dana has made converts of even the hardest clients.

0

Mr. Dana continued his prayer in an impassioned voice: "Thank you, God, for this wonderful opportunity to allow me to pass on new knowledge to help change all these beautiful people's lives. Thank you, God, for trusting me with these clients today."

Mr. Dana settled in at the podium and continued: "Addicts always practice praying. I know what a lot of you are thinking, 'Not another class on how important religion is in recovery . . . boring.' I'm not talking about religion, I'm talking about the Creator of the Creation. All of you in here had faith and practiced praying as an addict. You prayed all the time, every day. Unfortunately, you, the addict, prayed to a *Lower Power*. Let me give a few examples if I may.

"The addict is always praying that their dealer shows up on time, always praying that the dope is good, always praying that it weighs the right amount, always praying that they don't get busted for a DUI or drugs. Always praying they can make it home in time before their spouse or children come home, always praying that the 'penny slot' finally hits so they can get back the rent money. Over and over, day after day, year after year. Unfortunately, this is called 'misdirected prayer.' Make no mistakes, you all prayed in your addiction! All I am teaching you today is to simply manipulate your thoughts and energy to turn your prayers around."

Mr. Dana moved away from the podium and started walking around. "The addict begins to have faith in themselves by using the foundational tools we have previously discussed together. By using *Believing in Self* and *Not Doubting Self* together, and incorporating *Faith in Self*, you are creating *Spiritual Inertia*, and beginning to ignite a *Spiritual Fusion*, which develops into positive momentum.

This momentum propels you further forward into recovery. A rough definition of faith is 'to have confidence and trust.' All I ask is that you have this confidence and trust in yourself by knowing you are worth more. Eventually, you will develop faith in a *Higher Power*, rather than praying consistently to a Lower Power. For now, simply have faith in yourself. I mean, what do you all have to lose, anyway? Give it a shot. Fuck, if what I'm teaching you doesn't work, go back to praying to a Lower Power."

Slight laughter rippled around the classroom.

"In the Bible, in Matthew Fourteen, verse thirty-one, Jesus asks Peter to come and accompany Him on the water. As Peter begins to follow Jesus walking on the water, what happens?"

The class shouted, "Peter drowned, Peter sank."

Mr. Dana nodded his head and exclaimed, "That's right! Peter sank under the water. The reason why? Peter fucking *doubted* himself and lost *faith* in himself! Peter must have had the utmost faith in Jesus, or else why the hell would he follow Jesus onto the water in the first place? It is only when Peter realizes that he also was walking with Jesus on the water that he began to lose faith in himself, began to doubt himself, stopped believing in himself, and probably said to himself something like, 'What the fuck am I doing? I can't walk on water, I can't even swim. Holy shit!'"

The class cracked up.

Mr. Dana, becoming animated, continued, "Peter began to drown. The end result was Peter sinking below the water and Jesus saving Peter by grabbing him and saying, 'Oh ye of little faith.' Remember, Peter did not doubt Jesus. It was no big deal to see Jesus walking around on the water, as Jesus did all sorts of magic tricks every day.

"The addict knows how to pray . . . the wrong way! Practice the right way all day. Practice every day, but practice the opposite way that you did as an addict. Instead of asking for a jackpot at the casino, ask for a jackpot of feeling good. Pray for that. Rather than pray for better dope, pray for a better day. Pray to be free, pray all day for anything positive you desire. Begin to practice that.

"As you use these simple tools, remember that simple only means simple, it does not mean easy. Start believing in self, start not doubting oneself, have faith in self, and then add a Higher Power to pray to. Start asking God to help you in a good way. You are creating systemic synergy by using these three foundational tools. Realize you are slowly tearing down the old, addictive foundation. You *all* need to be conscious of this fact. You are doing this, I'm not. *You* are building a new foundation. Slowly."

Mr. Dana then started to walk out of the class, yelling over his shoulder, "Smoke break, twenty minutes. Don't be late coming back to class." And he was out the door.

Mr. Dana came back from the smoke break and once again sat at podium. "Alright, alright, settle down," he firmly stated. "I'm glad all of you came back to class and on time.

"Now, before the break, I talked about this new foundation and used the word *slowly*. I must emphasize the word *slowly* or *gradually*. All human beings live in a world of instant gratification, especially the addict. Using FaceTime, I can call and instantly see my daughter across the country. I can have a pizza cooked and delivered in ten minutes. Microwavable popcorn in thirty seconds. As an addict I can have a couple of shots of whisky and instantly be drunk. I can put a needle in my arm and nod out in the blink of an eye—instantaneously.

"Recovery does not work like that. Recovery is a slow, gradual process. You all need to trust in this slow process. It is not a light switch going off and on. Recovery is more like a dimmer switch slowly dialing up the brightness and beauty, not only inside yourself, but it brightens the beauty outside in your life as well. The quality and character of this 'dimmer switch' is that you can continue to dial it up forever.

"In recovery the question becomes, 'How hard am I willing to work to shine brighter and brighter?' Eventually, through practice, the *hard* becomes easy as these foundational tools become familiar and normal. They become instinctual, and we use them without any thought. Remember, recovery is an about face or complete change in direction. I'll give you a practical example. If you drive a car in the wrong direction and see you're getting lost, what do you do?"

Mr. Dana called on Marcos, who said, "Flip a birdie."

The class laughed along with Mr. Dana.

Marco then said, "Uh, U-turn?"

Mr. Dana nodded in agreement. "That's right. You make a simple U-turn. You turn around and begin to drive in the right direction. How do you know to turn around and go the right way? You ask directions, you consult Google maps, whatever. In recovery, when we are going the wrong way or we are lost, we must make a *You-Turn*. We must turn ourselves around. We ask and follow directions from someone who knows how to get to the destination. It is exactly the same thing. The car is lost, we make a U-turn. The human spirit is lost and continuing to go in the wrong direction, the addict must make a *You-Turn*. I know how to get there and am giving you all directions. Now, you make this You-Turn. You would do it in a car. Do it for yourselves.

"Class is over."

No Doubts

Mac: I arrived a bit late to class, and Mr. Dana was answering questions back and forth with the clients when I got there.

0

Mr. Dana turned to me between comments and said quickly and rather sternly, "If the clients can get here on time, and I, a sixty-five-year-old man who's had knee, hip, and back surgeries, can get here on time, then you have no excuse. Remember, the clients gave you permission to sit in on these classes and you need to respect that."

0

Mac: I thought, as much as Mr. Dana seemed so easygoing, there was no play time in the man when it came to the seriousness of his teachings. Looking back, I suddenly remembered what he had said in class long ago. He said, "This is the most serious thing you will ever do. Each of you is saving your life."

I took my usual seat behind Mr. Dana, vowing to be early to every class. This seat gave me a chance to observe the clients' facial expressions and body language to see what resonated and captivated them the most during these didactic lectures.

0

Without missing a beat, Mr. Dana continued. "As I was saying before I got distracted, as an addict, wherever I went

I was always so concerned and very worried about what other people thought of me. I was never comfortable inside my own skin. Regardless if I was loaded or not, I would walk into any situation, whether it be a family gathering, social situation, or a room filled with professionals, and give the impression of being secure and confident. The *real truth* is on the inside. I would be so scared. I would be shaking and lacking any self-confidence, with this dread reverberating down to my inner core. This fearful paralysis always gripped me so tight and never let up or let go.

"As all of you know, I have shared openly about being in the film business, and my point is that even on my best days on the set, when I succeeded so brilliantly and skillfully, I was always worried that someone with some sort of—I dunno, 'secret power'—could look inside me and they would *know* the *real truth* about me. Only after achieving recovery did I discover that this 'secret power' is called Real Truth, and the key was total transparency and allowing others to really see and know you.

"It was simple. In my addiction, the real truth was that I was a scared coward using drugs and alcohol to pretend to be someone I was not. I was a highly practiced, professional fraudster. Man, I was so good at pretending to be what I was not. It didn't matter, though, as I was always doubting myself. Making excuses and constantly manipulating the situation to erase any mistakes I made before getting caught.

"You see, the addict is always questioning themselves, even when making the right decisions. The constant, internal, negative dialogue is running nonstop, always questioning, always asking, 'Should I have done this? What if I did that? Why didn't I go about it this way? You fucked up again!'

47

"The addict is always full of doubts, even when successful. These doubts create un-stillness of thought and unease of self. These negative, internal manifestations are noticed by those who are on a 'higher level or plane of consciousness' and can see and feel Real Truth. To the onlooker or observer, it is obvious something is not centered 'within.' Regardless of whether the onlooker can quite pinpoint the problem, the onlooker knows instinctively that 'something is amiss' and there is something not quite right with the spirit.

"The beholder of these negative traits is always acting, always pretending on the outside that everything is cool and fine. On the inside the addict is under a constant, steady barrage of self-doubt as a result of this negative self-talk. The addict is always questioning self, asking self, 'Do they *know*?' Over and over, screaming, 'They *know*.' The question being asked is the doubt . . . 'Do they know I'm a liar? Do they know I'm crying inside? Do they know I'm so fucking scared? Do they know how guilty I am? Do they know I'm a worthless, hopeless, drug addict? Do they *know*?'

"This constant, never-ending, nagging doubt always results in further running from the Real Truth within. This doubt solidifies an already demoralizing lack of confidence in oneself. It is a losing situation. Whether it be a job interview, being in court, running into an old acquaintance, seeing your estranged spouse or children, the smell of fear and desperation is always present. It is the *souring* of the soul.

"The addict knows this, and the only way to rid themself of this personal stench and quieting the scream of their soul is to get higher! The louder the scream and worse the stench, the more an addict needs to consume—quickly.

That is the way an addict copes with the internal doubt, conflict, and fear. We run . . . we run to our addiction."

0

Mac: From my seat, observing the looks on the clients' faces, I was touched. Some of the individuals in the program were nodding their heads in agreement, some even had tears running down their cheeks. Mr. Dana continued to amaze me by always touching the clients in a gentle, caring way to make his point, using himself as the example. As Mr. Dana had told me on more than one occasion, "We are the keepers of the key to the lock. With respect, truth, and courtesy, the lock always opens. Remember, courtesy is the highest form of manipulation. Courtesy is one of God's purest tools."

I paid even more attention.

0

Mr. Dana was continuing, "When an addict embarks on the path of truth and begins to make any type of productive decision, it is irrelevant if those decisions result in mistakes. The addict learns it is okay to make mistakes. The addict in recovery is learning that most people are not judging and questioning those decisions, and if they are questioned on a mistake, it is not due to the fact that *they know*! There is nothing too *know* anymore except the truth about who you are today. You made a fucking mistake. Even I make mistakes, and you all know how close to perfect I am."

The class applauded and yelled in agreement.

"The recovering addict needs to understand and practice all day. Practice not to care about anyone judging them. Practice not caring if they don't meet expectations from others. That's their problem, not yours. The only one who should judge you and expect something from you is *you*. Every day, you need to look in the mirror and ask yourself one simple question: 'Did I do my best, did I give it my all?' When you can honestly say yes on a daily basis, you will realize you are beating your addiction. When you beat anything, it is called winning. Recognizing this every day is a little win. Every little win motivates you forward. When you know you are winning, you begin to develop self-confidence, self-worth, and self-esteem. The end result is that all the negative internal questioning *stops*.

"Judge yourself. Have expectations for yourself. If you don't meet your own expectations, work harder. Do good things for yourself. You need to have a chip on your shoulder. You need to prove to yourself every day that you are a winner.

"Remember, the addict who desires recovery has nothing to fear anymore and doesn't need to pretend they are something they are not. The true spirit within is learning not to doubt the decisions being made. The more the addict practices this, the more the doubts diminish.

"The final outcome over time is the empowerment of self and being proud of oneself. This self-nurturing is the reason we seek recovery. We are learning to put out the 'scream.' For the first time, the addict can now begin to understand how seeking a better, more positive way of life can be theirs, and the journey is actually just beginning. By believing in oneself and by refusing to doubt one's own self, the addict's spirit slowly starts to unlock from the inside the dark dungeon it has been trapped in.

"The soul, which has been confined and barely flickering since the addiction placed a stranglehold on its own self, begins to radiate energy. The recovering addict is now actually feeling the results of unlocking the powerful force within.

"That is *recovery*!

"Today, all of you are standing alone, isolated on the precipice of the highest cliff. There is no doubt that each and every one of you will fall off that cliff, get pushed off that cliff, or jump off that cliff as an addict. Those of you who implement what I am telling you will learn how to *fly* off that cliff. At one time I also stood on that harrowing edge, and as you can all witness, I learned to fly. All any of you need to do is follow me. The only requirement is to simply begin.

"Oh, yeah, I forget to tell all of you that any time I walk into a room today, I feel everyone should worry about what *I* think of *them*! As always, I am blessed, and thank you all for listening . . . class over."

Mental Discipline

Mac: Mr. Dana began his class with a remainder that everyone had to do their daily chores.

0

Mr. Dana: "Remember, when you don't do your chores the right way, you're not getting away with anything. You are not fooling the staff or me. Once again, what you are really doing is using your old way of thinking and your old addictive habits, cheating and fooling only yourself again. Learn to do the things you don't like to do to the very best of your ability. Give these things everything you have. Then, when you do something you really enjoy, it will be such a joy and pleasure."

Mr. Dana called on a client who had raised his hand. "Yes, Enrique?"

Enrique: "Mr. Dana, why do we got to do chores that has nothing to do with addiction?"

In a light, jovial manner, Mr. Dana replied, "Because you fucking live here."

The class cracked up.

Mr. Dana laughed as well and then said, "Alright, I want to talk about mental discipline. Discipline I describe as *forced habit*. I am *forcing* myself to do something. Minute by minute, hour by hour, day by day. In a simple way what I am doing and what is really going on is that I am training and forcing my mind to do something regardless of whether or not I want to do it.

"I wake up at five a.m. and get prepared to go to

work. It doesn't matter if I go to bed at eight p.m. or midnight, I get up at five a.m. I do this every day, without an alarm clock. My eyes pop open automatically and I get ready to go to work. Some mornings, it is freezing out, and I could easily roll over hold my wife in our nice warm bed and go back to sleep. What is going to happen? You really think anyone here is going to fire me?"

When the laughter died down, Mr. Dana continued, "Even though I am so thankful I get to come to work every day, do you all really think I want to get up at five a.m. every single day and see all the ugly faces of the staff?"

More laughter from the class.

"I said staff! I don't want any of you running to your counselors or therapists, crying that Mr. Dana said you were ugly."

More laughter and then Mr. Dana continued, "Most days I go to the gym. Do you really think I want to go to the gym after I get off work? C'mon, get real. The best part of going to the gym is leaving!

"My addictive nature tells me, 'You don't need the gym today. Don't go. You can work out twice as hard tomorrow. You deserve the rest. Think how hard you worked today.' If I allow that negative voice to control me, and I listen to it, I lose my freedom. I also know I will start to feel guilty for not doing what I needed to do. I force myself to go to the gym.

"Did you all hear what I said? I *force* myself to do something I don't want to do. It's a lot like doing chores in a program you don't want to do. Of course I would rather lay on the couch and watch TV after work. I refuse to listen to that voice. I force myself over and over, day by day, and what I am really doing is developing a positive habit through continual practice. This forced habit slowly becomes automatic. As I continue to force myself to do the things I don't like doing, I start ingraining this habit into my brain. This becomes *positive mental discipline*.

"I slowly see the payoffs or the benefits of my getting up for work in a fat paycheck. Or (gesturing to his pants) fitting into these skinny jeans by going to the gym."

The class laughed.

"The biggest change is removing the negative voice in my head. It is now a positive voice as I see the benefits of this mental discipline. I hear a different voice saying, 'Good job. You look fucking sexy.'" He flexed his biceps and the class laughed again.

"This positive habit has become automatic. If I don't go to work, I feel terrible. When I don't go to the gym, I feel sluggish and sinful. Why would I want to feel these harmful things and think negative thoughts about myself? I am in control of myself and am truly free. I do things that make me feel better, not worse. That's true freedom. The ability to choose things which help me to not hinder or harm my growth.

"All of you must be aware that you, the addict, possess this trait of mental discipline. The problem is that the addict uses this trait the wrong way. Think about it. The addict uses mental discipline in a negative way. For example, the addict has the mental discipline to be on time for a dealer. In fact, the truth is that the addict is never on time for the dealer—the addict is always early. Why? The fear of missing out. The addict will wait hours, which shows the addict possesses extreme patience. Now, that is strong, developed mental disciple. Imagine learning how to use that developed negative discipline the opposite way—the right way—to benefit yourself.

"For instance, getting to a job interview early. You might actually get the job. That's the payoff. How about picking your kids up on time from school? Instead of racing a hundred miles an hour from the casino and still being late. The benefit or payoff is that your kids are smiling rather than being upset. They are starting to believe in you again. What about using the negative discipline of extreme patience the positive way? Maybe you don't argue with your spouse as much. What's the payoff there? Perhaps you don't get as angry or frustrated waiting in line somewhere like the market, the doctor's office, or the bank. How many of you got all pissed off waiting at those places? You never, ever, fucking argued or got pissed off with your dealer for being half a day late. In fact, you thanked the dealer for being late."

The class laughed.

Mr. Dana asked, "What's that you said?"

Roberta called, "I never waited for a dealer or paid for any dope."

"Of course!" Mr. Dana replied. "Some of you worked for the cartel and had wheelbarrows of cocaine. I imagine a lot of you still have ice chests filled with millions of dollars buried on your estate overlooking the ocean in Malibu as well. Me, I wasn't a big-time dealer. All I wanted was a forty-dollar score.

More laughter, then Mr. Dana said, "You are all in this program today together, regardless of what a big shot you were in your addiction. Stop making excuses. The foundational tools are already ingrained inside the addict's psyche. But the addict is using those tools in reverse. The human being was not meant to destroy their own spirit. Your spirit is meant to 'empower' so it can continue to grow.

"By developing positive mental discipline through daily practice, forced habit, and training, the addict who desires recovery begins to feel inside themselves a ray of hope.

"That ray of hope begins to break through into the soul, and the addict starts to actually begin to feel better about themself. Now, that is a *huge* payoff.

"The addict in recovery actually starts *believing* in themself, has begun to stop *doubting* themself, and begins to have *faith* in themself. This new transformation starts to become noticeable to the person using these foundational tools.

"As I have said a thousand times before, these tools must be used repeatedly through daily practice all the time. Together, a symbiotic interaction takes hold and takes on a new form of powerful synergy, with the result being positive energy creating movement forward. With this synergy, the combined effect of the separate tools take on greater purpose. That purpose is the resolve to stay the course and, most importantly, allowing you to see the positive change you are creating. By feeling and creating better for yourself and within yourself, the addict will now begin to slowly correct old thoughts and habits into new ways of thinking.

"However, a new problem occurs. The problem is that if the addict uses and practices these tools daily, and then stops using these foundational tools, what occurs within is deep, negative emotions of guilt, along with the old addictive voice telling you all the negative reasons to stop this growth.

"Why does that happen? For the very basic reason that the addict has always had reasons, and listened to the old addictive voice make excuses, for not wanting recovery. Once you embark on this new path, you, the addict, now know the *real truth* of how to change for the better. The question is something you need to ask yourself at times of conflict between the old and the new. 'Why would I stop moving forward in recovery?' The answer is so clear: lack of forced habit.

"That is a key to continuing on the right path of recovery. Forcing yourself through mental discipline to understand that you deserve and want better for yourself.

You have decided through bouts of clarity that you do not want to feel the pain and guilt for any self-inflicted, negative thoughts or actions anymore. This is the real freedom in all of this. You have made the decision, no one else has forced you. That is pure liberation and a new stimulation. The addict in recovery starts to actually see a glimpse of the payoff: feeling better about themself.

"The addict starting recovery is so sick and tired of beating themself up and torturing those around them. The recovering addict wants to abandon all negative, self-inflicted, intrinsic—or extrinsic—events and actions to recalibrate their spirit and move forward.

"For the addict who wants recovery, who wants to develop new, moral habits and character, mental discipline is another weapon in the arsenal of foundational tools. Yes, I said *weapon*, because this is a war. Addiction and Recovery are at war within you. One side wants to kill you and one side wants to be free and alive.

"You all need to choose wisely. That is called 'The Art of Choosing.' One choice. All of you have only this one choice to make. The choice is whether you want to be a servant or a slave. However, either way, you all are going to serve!

"As always, thank you for listening to me. Class over."

Relentless Commitment

Mac: I observed Mr. Dana walking into class, talking to two new clients who had only entered the program straight from prison yesterday. He took these clients to a corner, and I overheard him talking to them.

0

Mr. Dana spoke in a low, normal tone. "I really understand that you don't respect yourselves. If you respected yourself, you would not have tried to kill yourself in your addiction. I truly understand that you don't respect others. If you did, you would not have put the people you care about in the position of worry and pain that you caused."

Mr. Dana's voice got firm and a bit louder. "However, you both will fucking respect *me,* as I have earned it here the past ten years. If you don't understand that, and allow your addiction to prevent you from respecting me, my staff, or the other clients, you can both pack your shit and get the fuck out. Either sit down quietly or leave now. If there is any type of disrespect toward the clients, my staff, or me, I will simply point to the gate and you're out. I am not threatening you, I am not warning you, I am promising you. Ask around. Mr. Dana don't break promises."

0

Mac: The two clients sat down very quietly. I remember when I first talked with Mr. Dana about how he was able to achieve unanimous cooperation from all the clients. Mr. Dana told me that most of the clients had at one time or another done some jail time. He also told me how much respect was a practice of survival in jail. He said to me that by throwing out those who were disrespecting others, it would strike a nerve subconsciously with all the clients, including the ones doing the disrespecting. Also, he told me that his ID on his lanyard, along with always 'dressing how he wanted to be addressed,' played an overall part in his achieving immediate respect due to the fact that, in the clients' mind, his image was one of an authority figure. Continuing, Mr. Dana said to me that, eventually, the respect he received came naturally to the clients. Rather than representing authority, he became relatable to the clients, establishing further trust and respect.

0

Mr. Dana came to the podium and began. "I apologize to all of you for the delay. I had a couple of clients who were a bit confused. I believe this confusion has been cleared up completely."

The class laughed.

Mr. Dana: "I want to talk to you about another foundational tool. This tool is *relentless commitment*. Let me talk about what that means. First, the term 'relentless.' To me this means being persistent and never giving up. Now let's look at 'commitment.' This simply means dedicated and making a firm decision to do something. Combined, these words simply mean, 'I will never give up, nothing will stop me in my quest for recovery.'

"Recovery needs to be a dedicated practice without wavering. Every second of every day, the addict must understand how important it is not to give up and not to stop pushing themselves. Not to give in to any mental temptation, such as doubt or a lack of discipline. The recovering addict must be unyielding in the commitment to win the toughest fight of their life. The fight to rid themself of years of negativity and the downward spiral of their life.

"This downward spiral is subtle and without any actual realization until it becomes almost too late. So fooled is the addict by this downward spiral based on deceptive rationalizations that when the addict finally hits the bottom of this spiral and looks up, it is even more demoralizing by the sudden *real truth* of how far they have fallen. In this dark depth known as rock bottom, the addict needs to begin the climb back up. That in itself can be very daunting, discouraging, and hopeless, especially with the addiction whispering words of destruction like 'failure' and 'quit.' This addictive voice has a beautiful, melodic, hypnotizing sound to the addict. I liken it to the sirens calling to Ulysses in Homer's *Odyssey*."

0

Mac: I sat there enthralled as Mr. Dana then gave a five-minute dissertation on the sirens and acted out Ulysses tied to the mast, relating Homer's story to the client's addiction. Mr. Dana always taught creatively and with a point relatable to the clients to expand the clients' knowledge.

0

Mr. Dana: "This is where the addict, anytime this 'voice of addiction' starts singing, reaches deep within and pulls out of the armory the weapon of *relentless commitment*, along with the other foundational tools, to take on this Herculean task. Only then can the addict think and feel about themselves in *really truthful* terms and have a desire to rid themself of their addictive sirens' song.

"The addict has always had that relentless

commitment to get up. I repeat, *to get up*. The addict is always getting up, and I use a boxing term, 'Never taking the ten-count' and not getting knocked out. It is the addict's relentless commitment to their addiction. The addict can lose their job, their spouse, their children, their home, their health and always get up for more. Always get up for more abuse from the ass-kicking, knock-down of addiction. Always justifying and saying, 'I am okay.' Making the most masterful, artistic excuses to others and, more importantly, believing those excuses themself. The addict is so committed to their personal death march.

"Unfortunately, sometimes the addict is knocked out for good. Sorry, let's not have any delusions—addicts do get knocked out. Stop believing your addiction's lies that tell you it can't be you. On average, illicit drug use led to almost one hundred thousand deaths last year. One hundred thousand! Those dead addicts were someone's child, brother, mother, or father. Imagine the horror. More people died from drugs than homicides. More people died from drugs than suicide or car accidents. That number continues to climb yearly, up over thirty percent year over year, according to the National Center for Drug Abuse. I don't make this shit up.

"Do you think any of those one hundred thousand who died last year thought it would be them? Fuck no! They listened to the magical voice of their addiction. Exactly as you all have been listening to it.

"The *real truth* is . . . addicts die. Yep, I said it. Addicts die. You all need to start understanding those two words go to together exactly like cake and ice cream, ham and cheese, fish and chips, peanut butter and jelly, butter and popcorn. Addicts die. Two very simple words that go together. Addicts die. Real truth.

"To stop that death happening to you, start

incorporating relentless commitment into your foundational tools war chest. As addicts, once again you have used that trait in reverse. Start using relentless commitment to achieve something meaningful, something along the lines of a better life! Using that relentless commitment creates a synergy and power inside the spirit, with the result being that the addict is getting restored. That godly power within can never be stopped, and I will prove that in a later class by using physics. Purity and light *always* wins out against the darkness which has infected your soul.

"These foundational tools take time. They are not instant. The problem you all face is that the society we all live in is so used to instant gratification. Whether it's ordering a pizza delivered to your home in fifteen minutes or talking to a family member across the globe through FaceTime. Instant, instant, always instant. We want it now! Put a needle in your arm . . . the result is instant. A couple quick drinks . . . the result is instant.

"Recovery is more subtle. In the Bible, Psalms Twenty-three, verse five says, 'My cup runneth over.' It is a process and so very gradual. Always keep that at the forefront of your mind. Your cup is your soul, and as it fills up and your spirit grows, you will need a bigger cup. I remember, growing up, when it would rain. My brother would put a frying pan or pot under the leaking roof. One single drop would hit the pan. A few seconds later, another drop. Then another drop. We would go to bed and when I woke up, the pan, spaghetti pot, or whatever would be full. I could never imagine how it could fill up overnight and overflow one drop at a time. Gradual. Over time. My cup overflows! That's recovery!"

The class clapped.

"Using these foundational tools is not an instant on-and-off light switch. It is more a dimmer switch going from dark to dialing up, slowly, gradually, into brightness. The thing about this recovery dimmer switch is that it continues to dial up your spirit brighter and brighter. This is known as *shining brightly* from within. Brightness in face and spirit, a glow, a vibe, powerful energy emanating from you. True empowerment of self and never ever letting go of yourself again.

"Incorporating these foundational tools all together, all the time, creates a *believing* in yourself, never *doubting* yourself, acquiring *faith* in self. Most importantly, learning to truly *know* yourself and who you are now becoming.

"As I have said previously, these foundational tools are a completely foreign language to the addict in recovery. Learn the language. Once the obsessive willingness of the addict to actually desire better of themself and want better in this life, the ongoing transformation will take hold, creating positive force, positive momentum, and positive change within. You all must begin to trust this gradual process. It is the opposite of how we all trusted our addiction to go into the tornado of the downward spiral of our addiction. That happened gradually as well. When I woke up, I asked myself, 'How the fuck did I end up way down here?'

"You see, addiction is a big, bad bully, and we all know what happens to a bully when they get confronted and smacked . . . the bully slinks away. Keep confronting your own personal addiction, and your addiction will slink away. All these steps must begin in conjunction with each other in a systemic fashion. Systemic means from the inside out."

Mr. Dana walked to the blackboard, wrote the word Hero and spoke to the class. "One of the definitions of a hero is someone who saves lives." Mr. Dana went back to the blackboard and, next to Hero he wrote Someone who saves lives.

Mr. Dana then asked, "Can anyone in the class name

me a hero?" He pointed to a client who had his hand up. "Bruno, give me an example of a hero."

Bruno replied, "I think a fire firefighter is a hero. Running into burning buildings to save babies and shit."

The class laughed.

Mr. Dana said to Bruno and the class, "Yes! That's a hero. Anyone else have a hero in mind?" Mr. Dana pointed to Shaniqua and said, "Go on, Ms. S, give me another example. You had your hand up."

Shaniqua said, "When my brother was in Iraq, he was with his squad, sitting in a circle having lunch. A terrorist from ISIS walked up in disguise and threw an explosive device in the middle of the group. My brother jumped up and threw his body on top of that bomb to protect the other men in his squad. The explosive device was a dud and didn't go off, thank God. My brother got a medal for saving his squad's life, even though it didn't go off. Praise God!"

The class erupted in applause.

Mr. Dana: "Wow. My God, thank you. That's such a deep story. It could have been so much worse. That is a real American hero." Mr. Dana then jumped up from the podium chair and said to the class as he put his finger to his lips, "Shhh. Shhh. No one move. I want you all to sit very still and don't make a sound, just listen."

He then put his hand to his ear, cupping it while walking to the door. "See how quiet it is?" He pointed to the glass doors leading to outside. "It's so quiet outside. Listen." He then yelled, scaring everyone and breaking the silence. "No one is fucking coming! I don't hear any firefighters or Marines coming to save you! No one is fucking coming! Tom Cruise and Mission Fucking Impossible ain't coming to save you. You are on your own. You need to be the hero of your life and save yourself, damn it! Be the hero of your life and save it from the enemy of addiction!"

In a very still classroom, and in a very passionate voice, Mr. Dana said, "I have told you repeatedly as a counselor and philosopher of addiction that it is not my job to save your life. My job is to instill new knowledge in you to teach you all how to save your own lives. To be the hero of your own life. It is yours and God's job to save your life. I don't need the pressure or stress. I'm busy saving my own life."

He stopped for a minute and then he simply said, "Great vibes all around. Thank you for trusting me and listening to me today. Class is over."

0

Mac: With that, once again Mr. Dana immediately walked out of the class.

Self-Motivation

Mac: Mr. Dana had told me last night over dinner that after today's final class on the foundational tools, he was going to start a series of new classes. He said he was taking his clients and classes to a higher level. In addition, he said he needed to challenge himself as well.

0

Mr. Dana begin his class by saying, "I describe *self-motivation* as the energy to drive one's own self toward personal dreams, ambitions, and desires. Self-motivation is the sheer force to keep going, regardless of any obstacles in front of oneself or any setbacks that are encountered. Self-motivation is the internal willpower to push forward towards one's goal. To acquire the mindset of a champion. Champions never quit. Champions get knocked down, not out. This is a fight for your life. There are no rules in this fight. Recovery versus addiction is a tough street fight. Addiction does not follow any rules, and your heart and mind have to be that of a champion. The champion's heart and mind say in unison, 'Nothing at all will ever stop me from reaching my goal and dreams. Nothing. Nothing will stop me! Regardless of how many times I get knocked down, I will not fail myself and succumb to my addiction and accept a life of personal negativity and spiritual rot. I will get up and pursue my dreams and goals.'

"What is behind self-motivation for the addict who desires recovery? Listen very closely. The motivation is to obtain a better life and to be free once again from any intrinsic or extrinsic, negative source which prevents you from being yourself and truly free. This *self-* freedom allows you to make your own choices and decisions in a positive way, regardless of the outcome.

"Again, the addict has always had and practiced self-motivation on a daily basis. I am only asking you to use this tool you have already perfected through repetition and daily practice. Use this tool you already possess in a positive way, the opposite way you previously used self-motivation during your addiction. Self-motivation is to enrich yourself in accomplishing anything you can imagine and propel you toward that goal. Self-motivation is not a tool meant to kill you in the pursuit of your addiction. Self-motivation is the internal force to make your life more meaningful and peaceful, allowing your own personal desires to come to fruition.

"The addict's daily motivation is to be 'all in' when it comes to their addiction and not allowing anything to get in the way. Again, your new self-motivation is to live, not die. Your new self-motivation is to obtain your dreams and the bountiful life God has guaranteed to each human spirit.

"Regardless of the addiction, whether it be sex, gambling, alcohol, or drugs, the addict wants to partake in the addiction immediately, as nothing comes before that addiction. I will give you a simple example. Say that the addict has children or a job. Anything the addict can do to rush through those daily responsibilities or commitments, the addict will do to the *least* of their ability. Any addict is highly self-motivated to rush through those obstacles. The addict knows that once those trivial things are taken care of—with the minimal amount of effort and time—the addict can move toward the one and only true goal . . . the addiction. The addict's only motivation is to indulge in the addiction as soon as possible. This negative self-motivation is an all-consuming thought, impulse, misdirected instinct to partake, or finding a way to achieve success as an addict by eventually reaching the goal of dying in the addiction. That is what any addict considers succeeding. Being in pursuit or taking part in the addiction without any distractions.

"Remember, the term self-motivation means nothing will get in the way of your desire to obtain your goal. If the addict does not have money, the motivation is to find a way of getting money through a perfected method or inventing a new method. The addict's arsenal relies heavily on the weaponry of cunning, lying, stealing, and deceit. The addict needs drugs. Again, the addict's motivation is to find a way to get some. If the addict is suffering in the full-blown clutches of addiction, the addict will always, always, *always* be motivated to find a way, regardless of the consequences or penalty, to enter into the addiction of choice as quickly as possible.

"The addict is always motivated to find a way and not be stopped. The addict's self-motivation always pushes them to always follow the path to the addiction and eventual self-destruction. The addict *always* finds a way. Talk about self-motivation!

"Now, if the addict could use this practice of negative self-motivation in a positive way, imagine the results. Let me tell you what the results are. It is the recovering addict who desires and begins looking for the gate to self-awareness to elevate their greatness. Self-motivation enables the recovering addict to be in touch with their own personal greatness, with the result being a better life. By willingly using this practiced, negative self-motivation in a positive manner, the recovering addict starts to achieve the principle of going back to the simple, basic ways of living and to find joy daily.

"That is the main reason or motivation to begin. It is simply daily joy earned by oneself.

"In the addiction, nothing stopped the addict. In recovery, once the process is employed, nothing will interfere with the recovering addict's self-motivation and the quest for 'the better,' to finally be able to step out of the shadows of the addictive life and re-enter the bright sunshine God provides. The dimming of your spirit in darkness and shadow that all addiction guarantees is not the human spirit's purpose.

"All individuals desire 'the better' for themselves, including addicts. Every fucking addict always wants better. Always. A better dope deal, better dope, a better pipe, better liquor, better sex, etc. etc. When the addict who embarks on this new path of recovery fully grasps and understands the real purpose and reason why using positive self-motivation will eventually lead to the desired results of obtaining 'the better,' the recovering addict begins to see what can be achieved by using this tool in a positive way. The recovering addict begins to practice—along with all the other foundational tools—self-motivation and has now taken a step toward 'the better.' The end result being better relationships with self, with family, a better quality of life, a chance at a better job, better able to understand themself.

"The new self-motivation is to be a real human being rather than a fraudulent, counterfeit actor always living in fear and pretending to be what they are not.

"Constantly practicing the first three foundational tools, along with this fourth foundational tool, leads to feeling better toward oneself. It is imperative that these foundational tools be used in conjunction with each other at all times in order to receive the optimum benefits and achieve recovery. These foundational tools will not work singularly, they must be used together to create positive strength. This positive momentum moves you in the direction you have always desired and wished for as an addict. Think how many times as an addict you screamed and cried out silently, wishing for help and any chance for positive change when you were in the darkest stages of despair during your addiction.

"The *real truth* is that you must be extremely open minded and aware that you are not being forced or coerced to do anything, you are not being lied to or being sold a false bill of goods. You all are simply being given a beautiful gift. This gift comes with one simple stipulation: Assembly Required by YOU!

"The end result is that your wish has come true.

"Thank you, class. You are all dismissed."

0

Mac: Mr. Dana left in such a hurry. I was hoping to see if he needed any help or to go over any material for his new classes starting tomorrow. Apparently not.

Summary of Foundational Tools

Once again, the whole purpose of understanding, incorporating, and achieving success with these Foundational Tools starts and ends with you, the user. The pure benefits are based on your own desire to desire again. That desire should be to end the enslavement of your addiction and obtain personal freedom through recovery. The amount of effort put into implementing these foundational tools will determine the overall success and outcome of your recovery. The real truth and bottom line is that the effort required is an investment in yourself. Ask yourself, "How much am I worth?"

Desiring recovery is the start of that investment, with the interest of that investment or payoff being a better life for you. That "divine dividend" continues to accrue throughout your lifetime. The overall result is creating a positive, residual effect on anyone associated with your life. That positive residual will continue to touch those in both personal and professional relationships.

It is important for you to realize that these foundational tools are not to be used strictly to obtain recovery and then discarded. Recovery is only the first step toward personal and spiritual evolution. The foundational tools have always been available and within your grasp. By using these foundational tools, you will create a simple spark to reignite your life.

In addition, these foundational tools must be practiced constantly and consistently to improve your daily life once recovery has been achieved. These foundational tools are meant to be used over the course of your lifetime to insure depth and quality of personal growth.

Like anything else, through repetition and repeated practice these foundational tools become a simple habit. The real effect and lasting beauty of using these foundational tools over and over with thorough daily practice is that they become instinctual. In our addiction, certain negative actions became instinctual. These negative instincts were employed without a thought and become second nature to preserve and insure the success of any addiction. You are now being taught to use these same foundational tools in a positive way through the "manipulation of energy," as I have demonstrated in the previous chapters.

With continued use, these foundational tools will promote, preserve, and insure a more desirous life experience for yourself and all who continue to gravitate into your presence. The powerful momentum you yourself have initiated and ignited internally will continue to grow and burn brighter, shining upon all who cross into your path. When you actually see that you alone are the cause of this catalyst and your own continued self-growth, this personal power you now possess cannot be stopped or extinguished.

I have previously discussed countless times that these foundational tools must be used together to create synergy. The combined effect is far greater than the effect of using them separately. These foundational tools do not and will not work alone. It must be a collaborative effect by all six foundational tools: belief, faith, no doubts, mental discipline, relentless commitment, and self-motivation.

The foundational tools act like gears operating any type of machine, the machine in this case being recovery. The foundational tools will not reach their full purpose without the meshing of these gears perfectly and in sync. The ultimate function of the foundational tools is to harmonize and balance your life. Creating harmony and balance in your

Dana Axelrod

life allows you to be free. Harmony and balance in your life allows you to use your imagination. Pure harmony and perfect balance in your life allows you to pursue. Perfect practice allows you to obtain your dreams.

Thank you.

—Mr. Dana

CLASSES

Revolution

Mac: Mr. Dana walked into class at a brisk pace and as usual seemed to be on a mission. As he was making his way to the podium, his class sat down and proceeded to give him their rapt attention. I had never seen anything less than the total obedience that clients and staff gave Mr. Dana during his classes. His classes were renowned for giving new knowledge based on people or events which had nothing to do with addiction until Mr. Dana wove them into his narrative.

Also present in this particular class were two case managers. They most likely were attending to improve on their own classroom skills. I was thinking what better way to enhance personal teaching skills than sitting in one of Mr. Dana's classes.

0

Mr. Dana began. "Good Afternoon and thank you for giving me another opportunity to instruct all of you on how to obtain a quality of life that God guarantees for each human being and, in addition, the conquering of your addiction.

"Of course, I thought I would give all of you a history lesson first. I want to start with talking about the American Revolution. Does anyone really know about that moment in our history? Ah, Ms. Jazz, you're the only one willing to take a chance? Please, go ahead."

Ms. Jazz: "I believe . . . wasn't it when the Americans fought the French for independence and Marie Antoinette said, 'Let them eat cake' and—?"

More than a few clients started to laugh uncontrollably. The laughter turned into contagious hilarity in the classroom. Mr. Dana did not say anything, he only gave a frown and a stern look while shaking his head. The laughter stopped rather quickly.

Ms. Jazz looked defeated and Mr. Dana said to her in a very gentle way, "I apologize, Ms. Jazz, on behalf of the ignorance of some of the *adults* in this room. In a group, it is easy to criticize. It is hard to have the courage to participate in front of others alone. Could you please continue? And remember what I have been teaching all of you. We do not allow others through negativity to control our feelings or our thoughts. *True freedom* is the ability to express our thoughts without fear or caring about what others think. We are *free*. That is what this class is all about. To be free.

Clearly embarrassed, Ms. Jazz stammered, "I th-th-think I was saying for America not to be ruled by the French? The Americans to make their own choices and gain freedom and independence from the French in a war?"

Mr. Dana: "Ms. Jazz, your facts are slightly off, yet the meaning is one hundred percent correct. You hit on the main concepts of what I want to discuss. Great, great job. Anyone else what to expand or share what you know about the Revolution? How about some of the fucking brilliant ones who were laughing? Not any of you? No? Okay, I'll go ahead."

0

Mac: Mr. Dana continued to amaze me. He always handled the endless situations—the bullshit which was always occurring in class or in the facility—in a "tutorial manner." He was always teaching. It seemed to me that he was making Ms. Jazz feel good about herself for sharing. In addition, he

*was putting the rude clients in their place through gentle
sarcasm and exposure of embarrassment. Any rude clients
would think twice about opening their mouths again.*

0

Mr. Dana: "Let's take a quick look at what Ms. Jazz shared.
She said the Revolution was fought for America to gain a
new freedom, along with independence from a ruling
country. That is correct.

"The word revolution means 'the overthrow of a
tyrant, dictatorship, or oppressive regime.' The only way
you can 'overthrow' or 'get rid of' is through violence. A
violent overthrow. That is what revolution expressly means:
violent overthrow.

"Now why do you suppose America wanted to
overthrow the country oppressing them? Oh, by the way,
Ms. Jazz, it wasn't France, it was Britain."

The class was very quiet, not a giggle.

Mr. Dana: "The fact is that the Americans wanted to
get rid of or overthrow the British. Why? It was due to the
fact that America was tired of being bullied, threatened,
always being told what they could or couldn't do. They were
tired of British law and the British ways of doing things.
America wanted to do it their way . . . an independent way
by being free of British dictatorship. The Americans were
not free, they were not happy, and they thought they could
do things better if they got rid of Britain.

"Now apply the word revolution to your addictions,
including negative thoughts, negative feelings, and negative
behaviors. Don't you all want to do things differently?
Aren't you all tired of being told what you can or cannot do?
Don't all of you want to be free and independent like
America wanted? What did America do? America went to

war!

"Learn from history. All of you have to start your own personal Revolutionary War. In other words, all of you have to *violently overthrow* this 'dictatorship' or 'tyrant' called addiction. This foreign ruler of addiction took away your hopes, dreams, and desires. This 'addictive dictatorship' which has controlled, oppressed, and suppressed all your freedoms needs to be overthrown. I am telling all of you that you need to start a personal Revolution in your mind. A *violent overthrow* of the dictatorial tyrant called addiction."

Mr. Dana pointed to his head. He walked to the blackboard and wrote REVOLUTION, and next to that word, in big letters, he wrote VIOLENT OVERTHROW.

Mr. Dana continued. "The reason I say 'violent' is that you have to *kill* your fucking addiction that rules over you and your entire life. The throne of your addiction sits in your mind." Again, he pointed to his head. "This Revolution has to be violent and instinctual. Whenever you think about your addiction, anytime you might want to indulge in your addiction, anytime you want to employ negativity in your life or in others' lives to pursue your addiction, you need to rise up, revolt, and fight to *kill* this controlling, repressive regime. That is what a revolution is all about. Rising up and fighting with everything you have inside of you. You need to say to yourself, 'Fuck no! NO!' Say this to yourself at all times. Violently denying and killing the thought, killing the words, killing the actions of addiction. This 'Fuck No' in the mind immediately and instinctually *is* the main weapon to use against addiction. Saying to yourself at all times, 'I am going to murder the dictator of addiction. I am going to *kill* this thought so there are no negative actions or behaviors.'

"You see, this is exactly how, during the French Revolution, the people rebelled against the tyrants! They chopped off the heads of Louie the Sixteenth and Marie Antoinette. The rebels *killed* those tyrants violently. You see, Ms. Jazz?" Mr. Dana nodded at Ms. Jazz.

"Ms. Jazz was right about *any* revolution. Regardless of whether it was the Russian, French, or American Revolution—or any revolution—the common denominator is an armed rebellion or uprising to violently overthrow an oppressive regime. That is the only way to gain new freedom and independence.

"All of you in here are Americans. You all celebrate the Fourth of July. Some of you think it only as a 'day off.' The Fourth of July is the celebration and remembrance of America's independence over the British. The early patriots demanded and fought with their lives for freedom and independence from the British tyrants. The early patriots put their lives on the line. Did you hear what I said? They put their *lives* on the line and were willing to die. And many did die. *There is a price you pay for freedom*! The price all of you are paying is to be here in this program to change your lives! All of you need to understand that to be free, you *must* make a choice. All of you have made a choice to stop being ruled by your addiction. All of you have made a choice that you are tired of being told what you can or cannot do by your addiction. You have all decided to be free. Wake the fuck up, all of you.

"*Your life is on the line*! This is *your* Revolutionary War against the oppression of your spirit. It is *your* war against the tyranny of addiction. When you get truly free from your tyrannical oppressors, that will become *your* personal Independence Day. Your clean date is independence and freedom! Mark that 'clean date' on your personal calendars, and you can all have your own Independence Day celebration.

"I am going to continue to use history and the

American Revolution as teaching examples. I will educate you with a powerful weapon each of you must develop for your own Revolution. When the American Revolutionary War started and all the patriots got together, was it to discuss a date and invite the British to drink tea and eat crumpets? Do you think these patriots got together and discussed the name of the British tailor because they liked their red coats? Fuck no. They wanted to *kill, murder, maim, destroy* the British, and they talked about ways to do it.

"Can you imagine the conversation when George Washington, Benjamin Franklin, and Thomas Jefferson all got together. What do you really think they talked about?" Mr. Dana continued in a cheery tone, "Do you think George Washington said, 'Hi, guys, I think this summer I am going to chop down another cherry tree.' Then Thomas Jefferson chimed in and said, 'Well, I'm going to plant some more corn and wheat on my farm.' Of course, Benjamin Franklin added to all this stimulating conversation by saying, 'I have nothing to do. I was thinking about putting a key on a kite and flying it in a lightning storm. What do you guys think?'

"Fuck NO! What they all said—and I know because I was there—" Mr. Dana had to stopped as the entire class cracked up. When the laughter died down somewhat, he continued. "They said, 'We are going to *kill* every last one of those fucking British! We will *not* stop until they are driven out of our country. Fuck the British. Kill our addiction! Kill the British. Fuck our addiction!' Say it with me!"

0

Mac: Mr. Dana was whipping the class into rioters!

0

The class yelled, "Fuck our addiction, kill our addiction."

Mr. Dana: "Louder! I can't hear you."

The class screamed, "Kill, Murder, Fuck, Kill our addiction, Fuck You, Addiction!!!"

Mr. Dana: "You hear that? You are putting revolution in the air! The American revolutionaries did it with their voices and actions. They screamed it from the rooftops. That was all anyone talked about. All of you learned in fifth grade how Paul Revere rode his horse, screaming the warning, 'The British are coming. The British are coming!' The early patriots had one united cause: killing the British and ruling America as an independent and free land."

Mr. Dana then pointed again to his head and heart while saying, "Your heart and mind. That is the land you're fighting for. Be a rebel and fight for these beautiful things God has freely given you.

"All of you in this class right now have to start fighting for freedom by putting your Revolution into the air. Start screaming out to yourself and all who will listen, 'I want recovery. I want to be independent and free from these old behaviors. I want to be free from these negative thoughts and habits. I want to be free from the dictatorship of addiction.'

"You need to become a rebel. The word rebel means 'violent resistance, to oppose, resist, and disobey authority.' The rebellion begins right fucking *now*!"

0

Mac: Mr. Dana was on a roll now. Speaking passionately and full of enthusiasm. The clients were engrossed, captivated.

O

Mr. Dana: "Countless times I walk by all you clients in the smoking area or recreation room. All I hear is the glamorization of your addiction. The constant blabbing, babble, blah-blah, talking of nothing. Talking of all 'the dirt' you all did in your addiction. Your addiction is not a badge of honor, it's a medal of failure. Stop bragging about failure and your misery. You all are keeping that tyrant alive. That's not 'fuck the addiction, kill the addiction.' That's keeping the dictator in power!"

Mr. Dana pantomimed choking an imaginary person. "To kill something, you have to take the oxygen out of it. Strangle murderously until it cannot breathe. I don't breathe air into something I want to kill. A lot of you keep breathing air into your addiction, giving life to your addiction. You need to violently overthrow those thoughts and words. STOP! Just stop talking about your addiction, don't keep it in power by continuing to breathe air into it. You need to start putting every breath into your recovery. Your life is on the line. You need to start putting recovery into the air and give it life. Not some of the time. Everyone, the staff, the delivery guy, everyone should hear, feel, and see recovery all the time from *all* of you, damn it.

"Nathan Hale said when he was about to be hung by the British, 'I regret that I have only one life to lose for my country.' This man is about to die and he said, 'I would give my life again for freedom!'

"Your tyrannical addiction is willing and trying to kill you at all times. Why aren't you willing to give everything you have for your freedom and independence?

"Okay, I need a break. We meet back here in twenty minutes. You all know the rule. Anyone who's late, no more smoke breaks."

When everyone was back in their seats, Mr. Dana started again. "Welcome back. I am really, really glad all of you came back on time. Oops, spoken too quickly. I just saw Case Manager Tommy coming in late." Laughing, Mr. Dana said, "I guess all of you no longer get smoke breaks."

The class loudly booed Case Manager Tommy.

Mr. Dana interrupted the boos. "Don't worry, you patriotic rebels. I won't hold you accountable for the staff's mistakes. Smoke and bathroom breaks still allowed." Then he said in a joking manner, "Mr. Tommy, I have been hearing that you want a shot at my title." Mr. Dana turned to the class and continued, "Case Manager Tommy, in all his classes, is always bragging how he is going to 'take the crown' from Mr. Dana."

The class erupted in howls and laughter

0

Mac: Mr. Dana was always opening up his classes with some sort of lightness or humor. I suppose this was his type of 'icebreaker.'

0

Mr. Dana, in a serious tone: "Let's continue this history lesson on the Revolutionary War, shall we? After the British were defeated in the American Revolution, what did the patriots do next? I mean, did they go home and chop wood or split logs for winter? Of course not. All the patriot leaders who rallied the rebels met together in Philadelphia. They met to decide the fate of this new, young country. They all sat down and wrote this thing called the Constitution."

Walking to the blackboard Mr. Dana wrote under the

84

word REVOLUTION the word CONSTITUTION. Under that line he wrote REVOLUTION = VIOLENT OVERTHROW and then CONSTITUTION = NEW set of principles or rules to live by.

Mr. Dana declared, "A *new* set of principles or rules. Why did the new patriots need a new set of rules to live by? Anybody want to guess? Alright, Mr. Rico, take a shot at it."

Rico: "Well, I think, as addicts, we all lived and followed a certain unwritten code or pattern of behavior. You've told us how as addicts we used different rules or principles to live by. Different rules as 'civilians,' as you call them, Mr. Dana. I imagine the patriots needed to all agree on a 'new' way to live free or a new direction to go after killing and destroying the British."

Mr. Dana: "Bravo! Bravo! Rico, you continue to impress me with how smart you are. And I don't impress easily. When the forefathers wrote the Constitution, they included what is known as the Bill of Rights. These 'Rights' laid out a new bold path, a new direction to live by. As Mr. Rico expressed, as addicts we had one set of rules. So now, as 'Victorious Freedom Fighters,' achieved by murdering your dictator of addiction, you all are going to need a *new* set of principles or rules to live by." He turned and wrote on the blackboard again: LIVE. "Look at the word 'live.' You need to start to *live* again by following and using a new set of rules and principles for this *new* path or *new* direction your spirit is now traveling on. You need your own *Bill of Rights*.

"All of you under the old dictatorship of addiction had what I call a 'Bill of Wrongs' that you used to *die* by. A 'Bill of Wrongs' followed by addicts perfectly. Now, we all need to establish a 'Bill of Rights' to live by. Hmmm . . . How do we design a Bill of Rights? Very, very

85

simple. We use 'substitution.'"

Mr. Dana again walked to the blackboard and wrote the word SUBSTITUTION. Then under SUBSTITUTION, Mr. Dana marked off two columns. One column he titled BILL OF WRONGS. At the top of the second column, he wrote BILL OF RIGHTS. Then he pointed to the "Bill of Wrongs" column and started to speak.

"Okay, I'm going to list a few items under the 'Bill of Wrongs.'" He wrote:

#1: LYING

#2: CHEATING

#3: DYING

Then Mr. Dana pointed to the column headed "Bill of Rights" and wrote:

SUBSTITUTE #1: TRUTH

SUBSTITUTE #2: HONESTY

SUBSTITUTE #3: LIVING

The class erupted in applause.

Mr. Dana looked at the entire class, laughing and nodding his head up and down. "I know, it's fucking brilliant if I do say myself. Anyway, see how easy this is? We simply use substitution. We substitute truth for lies. We substitute honesty for cheating. We *substitute* dying for *living*! And so forth.

"All of you make two columns and write your own personal 'Bill of Rights' or rules and *moral principles* to live by. We all can say, 'Revolution' and 'Constitution through Substitution.' And the last part is 'Evolution.' All of you memorize this. I'm going to give all of you my own personal history test later on. So remember: Revolution, Constitution by Substitution, Evolution."

Going to the blackboard, Mr. Dana added to his growing list of words and terms. Under SUBSTITUTION he wrote EVOLUTION = GROWTH AND DEVELOPMENT.

Mr. Dana: "Moving on from a history lesson to a science lesson, I will ask you, what is evolution? I'm going to tell you. Quite simply, evolution is the process of growth and development. By implementing these new principles you have achieved in your own Revolution through constant, *constant* daily practice, you will evolve. From an addict you will evolve into a new spiritual being. The *being* God meant you to be. This new path of self-awareness, along with self-discovery, will develop you mentally and spiritually. Spiritual growth—that's evolution. This growth is in all our DNA. God has programmed spiritual growth and spiritual development in each of us through our DNA. God has also programed in our DNA an undeniable thirst for more knowledge and a personal quest to keep moving forward in our lives rather than going backward.

"That is what I call 'the champion gene.' I would like all of you to look at all known civilizations that have always moved forward. According to Charles Darwin—he was born in 1809 and died in 1882—natural selection or evolution results when organisms evolve, making slight changes over time and adapting to living conditions that are best suited for sustainable living. All that means is that over time man finds suitable living space to live more productively.

"I'm not getting into Adam and Eve or other religious theories on the creation of man. I'll bypass all the arguments and simply start with known facts that are accepted by all religions. Man at one time starting living in caves. No one can deny that. There are countless examples of cave art, the Bible talks about living in caves, etc. So man lived in caves. No big deal. Then what happened? Do we all still live in caves? No. We evolved from living in caves to leaving the caves, and we began exploring the land. Any arguments here? None? Good. I'm glad all of us can agree on that.

"Now, use what I said earlier about a quest—which means searching for something important—and add in a thirst for knowledge, and eventually, man found themselves at the edge of Europe. Remember the song we all sang in third grade? In 1492, Columbus sailed the ocean blue. Do they still sing that song in third grade? They do? Great. From Europe, man used ships to get to North America over the sea."

Mr. Dana stopped. "I see Ms. Lilly has her hand up. Usually, you all know to save questions till the end of my thoughts; however, since Ms. Lilly is new, I'll allow hers. Yes, Ms. Lilly?"

Ms. Lilly: "I come from Iceland, and we know from maps, charts, and proven archeological facts that the Vikings came to North America five hundred years before the Europeans."

Mr. Dana: "Ms. Lilly, you are correct. However, I don't really want to get into Leif Eriksson and the Vikings. How Leif found North America before anyone. In fact, if my recollection is correct, Leif Eriksson landed on the coast of what is now Canada, at a place he called Vinland, in approximately 1010 AD. In addition, I believe Leif's father was Eric the Red, who left Iceland and discovered Greenland. Am I close to the truth of facts here, Ms. Lilly?"

Ms. Lilly, speechless and stunned: "Uh, um, yeah. You do know a lot about Norse history."

0

Mac: I looked around the class, and not too many clients were stunned by Mr. Dana knowing something about Norse history. It was a given that Mr. Dana could talk in depth about a myriad of topics. I was starting to understand Mr.

Dana Axelrod

*Dana's theory on DNA and a quest for knowledge. Mr. Dana
was a prime example of this "quest," as he was always
saying in class that he barely got out of high school.*

0

Mr. Dana continued: "I'm not getting into the Vikings or
how tribes crossed over from Siberia into Alaska. All of that
is irrelevant, as it only strengthens my point. That point is
that man was always exploring farther regions, evolving
man's knowledge and growing. Why? Why wasn't man
happy living in Ohio or along the East Coast? Why? It is due
to the fact man has the 'champion gene' that has been
programed into all DNA by God. God programmed a natural
curiosity in us to seek and move forward. The real issue is
that our addictions move us further away from this godly
programming."

Mr. Dana continued in an impassioned way: "Wagon
trains across America. Explorers. All of you, really think
about how *hard* it was exploring and moving across
America. It took years, births, deaths. There weren't any
roads, no air conditioning, No Hilton hotels for a shower. Do
you all think the wagon trains pulled into the drive-thru at
fucking Taco Bell?"

The class laughed.

"Talk about hardship. Why? Why do *hard* things?
Why push and push? The answer is that it's in man's DNA
to keep improving, to explore, to challenge, to *evolve*. And
our addiction cries out, 'Fuck it.' Your addiction screams,
'Ignore your truly pure, God-given instinct. You're fine
doing nothing and wasting your life.' That's the real reason
why each individual addict is plagued with guilt and shame
during the addiction. Addicts are going against God's *pure
planning*. Going against the *real truth* of God's programmed

DNA! And every addict knows it.

"Revolution to get to Evolution.

"Man flew to the fucking moon. Now man is going to Mars in 2031. Evolution.

"I want to finish up this class with this last bit. Each and every one of us, including me, has been lied to our entire lives. All of us. I remember, when I was growing up, all I heard from my teachers, from my parents, from all, from everyone was this big fucking lie, 'The sky's the limit. The sky is the limit. What a crock of shit. *The sky is limitless!* The only thing stopping us is this"—Mr. Dana points to his mind and his heart. "Class is over."

The room erupted in a pandemonium of applause!

Words

Mac: Mr. Dana came into class carrying a normal-sized box used for moving. He put it down next to the podium and then started class.

0

Mr. Dana called out in a firm voice, "Class, how you all doing?"

Various clients yelled out, "Fine," "Good," and "Great."

Mr. Dana now spoke in a really short, angry tone. "Okay, you all need to listen up. Fuck you. You suck. I can't stand any of you. In fact I hate all of you!"

0

Mac: I was in my usual seat behind Mr. Dana and facing the entire class. As I have often expressed before that I chose this seat so I could always observe the clients' body language and their faces during class and make my interpretation on what "hit home" and what "fell short." I didn't understand why Mr. Dana would say such things, and his words were entirely against his uplifting nature. I observed many of the clients had a look on their faces of bewilderment and disappointment. Others looked upset and confused. Quite a few looked at each other and shook their heads.

0

Mr. Dana spoke in a gentle voice. "Good morning. How many of you liked how I talked to you just now? How many of you didn't like the way I addressed you? And why?" Mr. Dana called on Tiffany.

In a quivering voice, Tiffany said, "I'm really upset. I don't know why you of all people would say those things to us."

Mr. Dana wrote on the blackboard the word UPSET. Then he asked, "Anyone else want to express themselves?"

A slew of hands shoot up.

"I want to hear from all of you," Mr. Dana said. He pointed to Andre.

Andre, in a pissed off manner, said, "I am really angry. I don't like being disrespected by anyone. That includes you, Mr. Dana!"

On the blackboard, under the word UPSET Mr. Dana wrote two more words: ANGRY and DISRESPECTED. Mr. Dana pointed to Charlotte.

"I only want to say I'm hurt," Charlotte said.

Mr. Dana went to the blackboard and wrote the word HURT, then he asked, "Anyone else want to express themselves?"

Denny: "I was really disappointed and felt betrayed, Mr. Dana. However, I have you as a case manager and know you, like, you know me. You have a plan and you're teaching us something. I just haven't figured it out yet."

Mr. Dana went to the blackboard and wrote two more words: DISAPPOINTED and BETRAYED. Then Mr. Dana began clapping his hands. "Bravo, bravo, Denny. You're one of my main men. You hit the nail on the head one hundred percent. I didn't call on the rest of you, but I'm sure the list of how I made you feel would only get longer on this blackboard.

"First, I want to apologize to anyone I might have insulted, made to feel bad, or brought out some feelings inside you that were bottled up from past negative arguments. My point is that words have such tremendous, creative power. Words can change how you feel about yourself or others in a heartbeat. Now, when you take any word and say that word with a certain tone or emotion, the word can be even more powerful."

Mr. Dana bent down and picked up his closed box, putting it on the podium.

Various clients in the room began to called out.

"Yo, Mr. Dana, what's in the box?"

"Hey, Mr. Dana, you bring us a present?"

"Mr. Dana, that snacks for all of us?"

Then the tone and comments began to change.

"Shut up, fool, pay attention."

"Who you telling shut up? You ain't my mother."

At that point, Mr. Dana stepped in. "Knock it the fuck off, all of you, and pay attention." He reached inside the box and pulled out a small, potted, flowering plant. "This beautiful plant is a daisy. Nothing special, it's simply a daisy. However, I'm asking all of you to forget it's a daisy and imagine this plant is my spirit when I was growing up. To understand what I am going to illustrate, you all must take this seriously. Now, remember, this plant is *me*." He put the plant on podium.

0

Mac: I'm watching the others and Mr. Dana. It is very quiet. Mr. Dana is circling the podium, with the plant sitting on top of the podium.

0

Mr. Dana suddenly screamed, about twelve inches from the daisy, "Fuck you! You suck. I can't stand you. I hate you!"

A few clients in class laughed a bit nervously. Others were staring at what they had just seen and heard from Mr. Dana.

Mr. Dana, sternly: "Remember, this plant represents my spirit when I was growing up. Take this seriously, damn it. This is not a joke. Why are any of you laughing at abuse directed at me? Growing up, these words were yelled at me on a daily basis. All day, every day. I am being completely open and honest with each of you. I am revealing something about myself.

"Now, some of you might have noticed that I used the *exact* same words yelling at my spirit that I yelled at all of you this morning." Mr. Dana pointed to the column of negative words he had written earlier. "Remember how you all felt when I yelled at you? How do you think my spirit felt being yelled at growing up? Think these words nurtured me in the right way? A beautiful way?"

Suddenly, Mr. Dana turned and moved once again to his spirit/daisy, this time stopping only about six inches away. Mr. Dana, yelled harshly and loudly as spit flew out his mouth onto the daisy/spirit, "You fucking piece of shit. I cannot even believe you are my son! You are so fucking *stupid*! You *cannot* be my son, you're so *ugly*!

The class was frozen, horrified.

Then Mr. Dana quickly spit on the daisy and smashed his fist right down on it, crushing the flower and a few of the petals fell off.

The class couldn't believe this. There was total silence in the room.

Mr. Dana continued the verbal abuse. "You are such an insult. You are *stuuuupid*!!! You are a *failure*. I don't want you to even breath my same air!" Suddenly, Mr. Dana lunged at the daisy and threw it across the classroom.

The class, in entirety, groaned. A few clients were crying quietly.

Then Mr. Dana walked across the room, picked up the plant, and took the broken daisy in its cracked pot back to the podium. "My spirit will still grow. But it will grow crooked. It will grow broken. It will 'get by' and survive. As I told all of you previously, as addicts we all know how to 'get by' and survive. Unfortunately, that is not what God intended for our spirits.

"Now, imagine how my spirit feels. Anyone want to share?"

The entire class had their hands up

Roxy, starting to sob: "My parents used to yell at me m-my whole, entire"—crying now—"life when I was growing up. They made me feel so small."

Damian, shaking his head: "Damn, Mr. Dana. Damn. Damn, damn, damn. How did you know?"

Reggie: "You ain't alone."

Mr. Dana then said, very gently, "Yeah, a lot of us have more in common than we think. However, I know how to fix this crushed, broken spirit.

"Now really, really imagine this is *your* spirit and it has grown up a bit. Imagine that this spirit is now sixteen. It has been treated this way by almost everyone for sixteen years. Imagine, if you can, what this spirit says or *always* thinks and feels about itself."

Mr. Dana pulled the daisy/spirit right up to his face, right in front of his lips, and spoke. "Daisy/Spirit says to itself, 'You are worthless. You are a piece of shit. You can't do anything right. You are ugly. No one wants you around. You are a failure.' Internally, these thoughts and feelings go on and on. Day by day. Growing ever larger, harsher, harder.

"However, I told all of you I know how to fix this

immediately." Mr. Dana went into his box and pulled out a baggie. He poured the white contents onto the spirit. "Look, I'm putting cocaine all over the plant. Let me make sure I mix it really well with the soil. This cocaine is great fertilizer."

The class laughed.

Mr. Dana then reached into the box and pulled out a bottle of vodka. Speaking soothingly, he said, "You like that cocaine, don't you, Spirit? Here, have some of this as well." Mr. Dana poured the vodka all over the spirit/daisy. "You're thirsty, aren't you? Tastes good. Yum. How do you feel now, Spirit?"

Mr. Dana put his ear to the daisy. "What's that you say? You don't feel anything at all anymore. What? You don't care about anything, not even yourself? What? Sure, I'll give you more . . . and more . . . and more."

Mr. Dana: "And so it goes."

Mr. Dana put the broken, drunk, drugged-out plant back into the box and pulled out a big, beautiful, potted, fully flowered, bright-colored daisy. With his ear right next to the new daisy, he started talking in a gentle, soothing voice. "What? Yes, I agree, you're beautiful. What? Of course you should be proud of yourself. What? Yes, I know you're not the same as you were growing up. Of course, I agree totally. You are most certainly really alive and really thriving. What? Yes, you *have* changed for the better, and God loves you. You now love yourself? That's such a beautiful blessing."

Mr. Dana turned from the daisy, looked right at the class, and said, "If you love yourself, you will never want to harm or kill yourself with addiction.

"The creative power of your words can fill each of you with gloom, or the words can doom you and your future. Just as I taught you in the class about revolution. You must stop keeping old thoughts, old actions, and old feelings alive by saying the same old words you used in your addiction. I have previously taught you that those words are a foreign language. Forget how to speak that language of heartbreak, misery, and failure. Use the creative energy of new words. Use your words to propel you forward where you want to go and how you want to feel about yourself.

"Words are 'predictors.' If any of you really want to know where you're headed in six months or a year, listen to your words. What are you saying about yourself right now? Do you really think you will be feeling differently about yourself in the future if you're talking about yourself in the same negative way? What you are saying and thinking about yourself must be done with 'the knowing' that your words matter all the time. Matter *every* time. Start telling yourself wonderful things. Tell yourself what direction you want to head in and make it matter.

"You don't have to listen and believe me all the time. I don't know *everything*."

The class and Mr. Dana all laughed.

Mr. Dana: "No, seriously. If I don't know everything . . . but God *does*. Let's look at the Old Testament. You've all heard of the city of Jericho, haven't you?"

A few clients said yes. A few clients shook their heads no.

Mr. Dana continued in a moderate, easygoing tone. "Okay, some do, some don't. How about the song "The Walls Come Tumblin' Down" by U2? Now I have your attention. I see a majority nodding their heads up and down. You all like the group U2, I see. That song is about the city of Jericho. Jericho was a walled city. Huge walls. I mean *massive* walls encompassed the whole city. The walls were impenetrable. Now, Joshua and the Hebrews wanted to take this city. The problem was that they had no way to make 'the walls come tumbling down.' I mean, those walls were massively thick and really high.

"In Joshua, Chapter Six, verses fifteen through twenty, the Lord says to Joshua something like this: 'Joshua, all you got to do is march around the city for seven days with your people and blow these horns. That's it. Just take your three hundred followers, march around the city for seven days blowing these horns, and *I will do the rest*.' Now, Joshua trusts the Lord, so he believes, has faith, and agrees, even though Joshua is thinking something like, 'Just blow these horns? The Lord must be crazy!'

The class laughed.

0

Mac: Mr. Dana was an amazing storyteller. Always acting out the parts and using his voice in a very modulating way. Mr. Dana's voice would get loud, soft, humorous. It always kept not only the class entranced, but it kept my attention as well.

0

Mr. Dana: "As Joshua was gathering up these big horns, the Lord said one more thing to Joshua. 'Look, Josh, there's one more thing—'

"Of course, Joshua was probably thinking, 'Fuck, I knew there was a catch to all this. Blowing horns for seven days isn't going to work alone.' He thought something like that. I was there, of course. I'm not a freaking mind reader, though."

The class laughed again before Mr. Dana continued, "Anyway, the Lord continues talking to Joshua and says,

'The one thing, the key to all of this, is you. Joshua, you have to make sure that everyone in your group, all three hundred, don't say a word. Not one word. No one can utter anything. Just blow the horns.'

"So, after seven days of blowing the horns, the 'walls came tumbling down.' Why am I telling you this story, some of you might wonder? Because the Lord God knew that when you get three hundred people marching in the desert and nothing immediately happens, people are going to start fucking complaining."

0

Mac: Mr. Dana started pretending to be different Hebrews marching on Jericho.

0

Hebrew #1: "My lips are chapped from blowing this fucking horn. This ain't going to work."

Hebrew #2: "Your lips are chapped? I'm fucking thirsty with all this dust in my mouth. We haven't stopped for half a day."

Hebrew #3: "Thirsty? Shit, I'm getting blisters on my feet. These sandals suck."

Hebrew #4: "All of you shut the fuck up! My underwear's been going up my ass all day and I've got a hell of a rash!"

The class erupted in laughter.

Mr. Dana laughingly said, "You see, God knew that people complain. God knew if people complain then nothing gets done. Nothing gets done and complaints spread like infections. So God showed all the Hebrews that if you want something, blow your horn and don't complain."

99

Janice: "Mr. Dana, I understand the story and about not complaining. But I don't have a horn to blow."

A chorus of clients: "Yeah, we don't have a horn."

Mr. Dana: "The horn represents your voice. When you wake up in the morning, stop bitching. Use your horn—your voice—to thank God for another beautiful day. Stop complaining. It's not only affecting you and your day, it infects everyone else around you. You all think you got problems, huh? I'm gonna tell you who's got a problem. The person who did not wake up today and is *dead*. They've got a big problem. They're fuckin' *dead* and don't even know they're *dead*. That's a big problem.

"According to the World Health Organization, a hundred and sixty-seven thousand people die every day on earth. One hundred and sixty-seven thousand! You all ain't one of them today. Be grateful God has blessed you one more day, and blow your horn. Thank you, God! One more day. Blow that horn. I've got news for all of you. When God tells me my time is up—" He pointed to one client, then another client, another, and another. "I'm gonna tell God, 'Give me *his* problem, *her* problems, shit, I'll take the whole class's problems all together.'"

He pointed to the whole class and then down to the ground. "You all get in that fucking hole." He pointed his hands upward. "Thank you, God, for this day! I'm blowing my horn. Thank you, God!"

The class exploded with applause.

Mr. Dana: "I have at one time or another asked most of you in this program one simple question. I have been asking this exact same question since I first started working here. I even asked others outside the program the same question. Whenever I see someone in the morning, I ask them this simple question: 'How do you feel?' That's all. How do you feel? The number one answer every time—or nine out of ten times—is always the same. 'Tired.' It doesn't matter if the person answering the question is young or old. It doesn't matter if that person stayed up all night or slept for a week. The answer is always the same. 'Tired.' Do you know why? Because people have programmed this word into their psyche. They might not be tired, they might be sleepy, foggy, exhausted, or don't really know how they fucking feel. But they have programed this word into their brains.

"Now, class, when someone says they're tired, how do you think they're going to feel all day?"

The class shouted in unison: "Tired."

Excited, Mr. Dana said, "Exactly. Unfortunately, they have talked themselves again into being tired. Now, if you can talk yourself into being tired, don't you think you can master the *power of the word* and talk yourself into being awake? Happy? Excited, great, successful, blessed? Start self-hypnotizing your speech to use the power of words to work for you, not against you. Start self-hypnotizing yourself and tell yourself how you want things to be in six months to a year. Don't wait for tomorrow, start right fucking now thinking really good, positive, beautiful things about yourself."

Mr. Dana continued, "The power of words. Proverbs, Chapter Thirteen, verse two says, 'A man shall eat good by the fruit of his mouth.' Think about that. If you want to eat good, say good things.

"It is not all your fault. It's also the fault of a lot of the case managers, therapists, and staff. The entire staff is always using these negative, defeatist words like 'self-sabotage' and 'fear of success.' Fear of success! My God, how many of you have ever achieved success?" He looked around.

"Success is nothing to be scared of. Repeated failure or failing to even try, now that is scary. That is what addicts do. They find ways to be scared and not even try. Anyone who achieves any success realizes it is due to their individual actions. That isn't fear, it's being exuberant. It builds up self-worth and self-value. Remember that when you get a job, when you get a raise, when you get a promotion, the common denominator is *you*. You did that. That isn't scary. All of you, I want you to think about the scariest place you have been in your addiction. Anyone want to share the scariest moments in their addiction?"

Tomeka: "I remember being in a motel room with, like, six guys. I didn't even know them. I wanted drugs. That . . . sheesh, that was *scary*!"

Ronnie: "I remember when I sold our car, emptied out my wife's and my bank account to bet on a horse. I got a big tip. It was thousands of dollars. I lost. I remember taking a bus home then hitchhiking. Walking into my house and looking at my wife and telling her how I fucked up again. That was the all-time *scariest* situation I have ever been in. And I've been to Iraq!"

Mr. Dana: "Oh my god. Thank you both. All of us have been in scary shit as addicts. You think going and interviewing for a job or meeting your spouse's parents is scary? You all know scary. Achieving success is not something to fear. This is all the staff's fault. Look at the words that control us in recovery.

"I'll give you another example: the 'pink cloud.' For anyone who doesn't know what the pink cloud is, I'll tell you. It's a theory that when you get clean, after about forty-five days, you feel really good and then you hit this so called 'pink cloud' and come crashing back to reality. I refuse to allow something like a word to dictate how I *should* feel. Fuck the pink cloud. After forty-five days, I *flew* through the pink cloud. I be lying if I ain't still flying. I haven't come down. In my recovery, I keep going farther and farther up!"

The class clapped.

Mr. Dana: "Class, can I count on all of you to be *really truthful*? I want to end class on the power of words. You must use and be in the *real truth*."

The class all yelled, "Yes."

Mr. Dana: "Okay, good. I knew I could count on all of you. In our addiction, how many of you ever called, asked, or said to someone, anyone something like this? 'Hey, I need some shit,' or 'I got some good shit,' or 'Do you know where I can get some shit?' Something along those lines. Show of hands, please.

"Wow, almost all of you." Mr. Dana wrote on blackboard the word SHIT. Then he said, "Remember, you all said *real truth*. How many said something like, 'I need some dope. You got some dope? Can you get some dope?' Show of hands, please.

"Hmm, about half of you. Okay, how about something like this? 'I'm dope sick, I need some shit or I'm gonna be dope sick.' Show of hands please.

"Better. About three quarters of the class."

On the blackboard, under the word SHIT, Mr. Dana wrote the word DOPE.

Mr. Dana: "How many of you ever said something like, 'I got fucked up last night,' or 'I want to get fucked up, let's get fucked up?' Something like that? Again, a show of hands, please.

"Really? All of you. That's honest."

Mr. Dana wrote FUCKED UP under DOPE.

Mr. Dana: "How many of you ever said, 'Yeah, I got wasted last night.' Or 'I want to get wasted, let's get wasted,' or 'Man, was I fucking *wasted*.'

"Same thing, show of hands, please. Impressive, almost all of you again." Mr. Dana went to the blackboard and added the word WASTED. Then he turned and addressed the class in a very direct manner. "Words and their power. Words can hurt us, as I have shown all of you today. The power of words can make us feel really, really good, as well.

"The one last thing I want to show all of you is that words are 'predictors,' meaning they predict what we want and they predict our future as well. Let me prove how powerful all your words can really be."

Mr. Dana pointed to the blackboard and said, while pointing, "Shit. You all asked for shit and got into a world of shit. You all asked for dope and now are the fucking dopes. You all said you wanted to get fucked up. Now you have fucked your life up"—still pointing—"and finally, all of you wanted to get wasted. You all have *wasted* your lives and, more importantly, wasted the most precious gift of all . . . your *time*.

"Do you all now see the power of the words you were using? Today, instead of asking for shit, use the power of words to ask for things of *value*. Never again ask for dope. Today, right now, start asking for *hope to cope*. Instead of asking for or using words to get fucked up, start practicing and using your words for 'I am growing up' and 'I am standing up.' And finally, instead of wasting your lives, start using self-hypnosis to *enrich* your lives. Have a *meaningful* life.

"The power of words. Make *your* words empower *your* direction in life.

"That is all. Class dismissed."

Everyone in the class stood and clapped and cheered.

0

Mac: In the empty classroom, I was left alone and thinking. Thinking about the meaningful teachings I had just been witnessing.

104

Wants Versus Needs

Mac: I arrived at class a bit early and sat in my usual chair against the wall behind the podium. Since I had become more comfortable and somewhat known to the clients as a result of attending Mr. Dana's classes weekly, I began alerting the clients that Mr. Dana was in the accounting department and would be a few minutes late.

As I began some bantering with the clients, Mr. Dana came bounding through the door with more exuberance and energy than usual. His presence always energized everyone, everywhere. This was especially true in a closed setting like this class. Today, though, he seemed more electric, more on fire—if that were humanly possible. As Mr. Dana got to the podium, the usual smattering of applause and respectful yelping from the twenty-five or so greeted him.

0

Mr. Dana began laughing in a very uplifting, spirited voice that was bordering on unbridled excitement. "I'm really, really sorry I'm a bit late today, however, it's such a beautiful day and I have truly been blessed. It's Friday and I'm off after this class. Maybe I'll even cut class from ninety minutes to thirty—"

A loud chorus of boos rippled across the classroom.

"I have an extra-long weekend since Monday's a holiday. Think how great recovery truly is; I get paid to have Monday off . . . a three-day holiday. Woo-hoo!

"I want all of you to be really honest. Can any of you truly remember if you ever had a day off, a paid holiday, or a vacation in your addiction? You all need to remind yourself of this very fact. My guess is none of you ever did. Addiction may have first started out as a vacation or holiday . . . but your destination was Hell! Keep remembering the pain you caused to yourself and the pain you were responsible for in others.

"Remember, recovery is about being brutal, honest, and really truthful to yourself. I don't expect anyone in here to be a hundred percent truthful with me, your therapist, or those closest around you. Why would you be totally truthful or trusting to me? Let me tell why you can't. It's actually quite simple. In your addiction you could not even tell yourself the truth. You could not even be honest with yourself. Think how many times you looked in the mirror with your face all sucked up. What did you say to yourself? 'Man, look at my cheekbones. I look like a model.'"

Mr. Dana waited for the laughter to die down and then he continued, "Or your face was all bloated and your eyes were red, and you told yourself, 'A little Visine and a shower and I'll be fine.' You could never stand and face yourself with the real truth.

"However, if you really want lasting recovery, you *must* face yourself and be honest by telling yourself the truth. What is the identical quote every NA and AA chip has embossed on it? None of you know? Really? You all have chips, even if it is a newcomer chip, and you all don't know? On every chips it says, 'To Thine Own Self Be True.' Think about that quote."

Getting passionate, Mr. Dana exclaimed, "Shakespeare wrote that. He is considered to be one of the greatest writers about man and the human condition. What Shakespeare is saying is, 'Tell yourself the fucking truth!'"

Now, sounding exhausted, Mr. Dana said, "Man, when I think back about how many times I wished I didn't have to get up and go score . . . Waking up really early or coming home really late. That was especially true on holidays, which were the worst. We were always lying to our families. All of us had to work like slaves on Christmas, New Year's, Thanksgiving, every holiday, without any holiday pay. Even when we were going on vacation and then cut the vacation short. Why was our vacation cut short? We ran out of fucking dope!

"Lying to our families and making some elaborate excuse why the vacation was abruptly ended. Lying even more by saying, 'I will make it up to all of you.' No peace of mind, no time ever, ever off. Our addiction was a full time, twenty-four/seven job. Our addiction was a tyrannical taskmaster. Always making us grind, sweat, filling each of us with panic, despair, and worry. Addiction is the original boss from Hell.

"But I digress. I don't know how I went from such a blessed day into a lecture on the *real truth* of addiction. Ha-ha."

0

Mac: It was masterful. That's why Mr. Dana is a magician. He came into class talking about his blessings, days off, being upbeat, then he started shifting gears seamlessly and began his teachings of the day on "Real Truth to Self," using reality and our past experiences. He then dropped a velvet hammer to beat our psyche into honest submission. That is the beauty and the gift he has. He reels all of the clients in and then delivers the fatal knockout blow. Pow! The clients never see the punch coming.

After knowing and shadowing Mr. Dana, I listened, studied, and learned. Now I knew he was just getting started on his carefully planned lesson for the day. I doubt if he was really in the accounting office it all. The way I view Mr.

Dana is that he plays the Pied Piper and the clients follow him out of their misery of addiction into the Promised Land of Recovery.

He continued to weave his good fortune and blessings in a personal way as he continued to speak.

0

Mr. Dana: "I'm going to tell you what's even more beautiful about today. It's payday! The accounting department has been making mistakes on my checks for months. They finally issued me a check with all of my accrued, unpaid salary for the last three months. God is so great. I love my life today. I used to sit in those very same seats—" Mr. Dana pointed to the clients sitting in the classroom and said, "I want all of you to imagine my life today."

0

Mac: Mr. Dana was a great maestro, always changing his tone of voice. Now he was using a more conspiratorial tone and in a low whisper, enticing the clients to feel they were all in together on a secret.

0

Mr. Dana: "Imagine getting paid for what I do." Putting his finger to his lips, he looked around. "Shhh, no one knows." With a wink and a laugh, he said, "Please don't let anyone in management know I would do this for free!"

Changing his voice again like a virtuoso, soloing at a keyboard, his tone was now intense and passionate. With his finger to his lips, Mr. Dana began waving his check around, looking at it, acting shocked as if he disbelieved how much his check was for. Then he said, "I really *want* to go to the casino, I *want* to leave for Vegas right now! I *want* to play blackjack, I *want* to play roulette, I *want* to play craps!" He paused then continued in a more serious, hushed tone, "I *need* to pay my rent. I *want* to gamble . . . I *need* to pay my rent."

Mr. Dana made it sound like a hypnotic mantra. "*Want* (pause) *need. Need* (pause) *want. Want* (pause) *need.* He looked at everyone in the class and, using his hands as scales, repeated the words back and forth. He kept the mantra going. "*Want* to gamble . . . *Need* to pay the rent . . . *Want* to gamble . . . *Need* to pay the rent . . . *Want* to gamble . . . *Need* to pay the rent."

This went on for a few moments and suddenly, Mr. Dana asked all the clients, "What do you think I'm going to do?"

A majority of the class shouted, "Pay your rent!"

One or two of the new clients yelled, "Gamble!"

0

Mac: Apparently, those who said "gamble" were very new to the program and recovery, as they had not yet fallen under Mr. Dana's cosmic spell of productive and positive change. Eventually, they too would become "believers."

0

In a serious tone, Mr. Dana then asked, "Do you know the difference between children and adults? Children do what they *want* to do; adults do what they *need* to do. Do you know the difference between addicts and adults? The addict does what he *wants* to do. The adult does what he *needs* to do. I *want* a Ferrari; I *need* a cheap car to get to work on time, I *need* to save money to pay for my kid's braces. I *want* a house in Malibu overlooking the ocean; I *need* a roof over my head for my children and myself.

Wants versus *Needs*. Adults do what they *need* to do. If adults continue to take care of their *needs*, they might get to do what they *want*. Start doing what you *need* to do, not what you *want* to do. You *need* to be responsible. You *need* to take care of your family. You *need* to stop using drugs."

The classroom was quiet and still.

Mr. Dana continued, "You all know me. There is no play in Mr. Dana. Only *real truth*. This is the most serious thing you will ever do . . . to save your life. Some of you are under the misconception that it is Mr. Dana's job to save your life. Wrong! It is my job to educate you on positive change. I'm busy saving my own life. It's your job and God's job to save *your* life.

"I'm gonna be quite frank with all of you. I really *want* to get high. I *want* to have a few drinks, snort a couple lines. I *need* to stay sober, my family *needs* me, my family is counting on me, all of you are counting on me, and my spirit is counting on me.

"Needs versus *Wants*."

With that, Mr. Dana walked out of the classroom and was gone—followed by the usual applause.

Affirmations

Mac: Mr. Dana walked into class, greeting several clients on the way to the podium. Mr. Dana was carrying a small, plastic grocery bag. I always found it interesting whenever he brought something like a box or a bag into the class. I have come to expect some type of "visual" demonstration to go along with his lectures.

0

Mr. Dana: "Good morning, all of you. I hope you're all doing wonderfully. Before I get started this morning. I want to once again thank you for coming to class on time and not fucking around. It shows me you want recovery. Today, I would like to continue to go further in depth on one aspect of last week's class. Power of Words. A quick review from last week is simply how important words are when using them to communicate with others or using words on ourselves. Words have the power to hurt you or heal you, as I discussed last week. Please, in today's class, continue to follow the thread of that topic and its theme.

"Today, I want to discuss the meaning of affirmations and how using affirmations can enhance the power of words on a personal level. I think we need to all be clear on definition of the word 'affirmation.' We need to all understand and be and united in the context I'm using it in for the purpose of this lecture. Anyone know what an affirmation is?

"Go ahead, Natalie, and then Julian."

Natalie: "My therapist says it is telling yourself good

111

things and that I should do this every day."

Mr. Dana: "Well, you aren't wrong. That would be using 'positive affirmations.' Where and when did your therapist tell you to practice these 'positive affirmations'?"

Natalie: "She said to do them every morning in the mirror."

Mr. Dana: "Ok. Would you mind reciting a few to the class so we get an idea of what you mean?"

Natalie: "No problem. My therapist gave me a list." Natalie flipped pages in her notebook. "Okay, here it is. The first one is, 'I am beautiful.'" She read a few more from her list: "I am successful, I am confident, I am—"

Mr. Dana cut her off. "Thank you, Natalie. I stopped you for one reason. I want you to put the list you're holding back in your notebook. Please, if you don't mind, can you do a few more for us without reading that sheet of paper?"

There was a slight hesitation in her voice as Natalie said, "Mr. Dana, I really don't feel comfortable without the list. I can't do them on my own. I can't think of any."

Mr. Dana: "No problem. And thanks for sharing."

The class clapped.

0

Mac: I have noticed that Mr. Dana always asks permission for a client to share, as well as never pointing out if a client is wrong. In addition, he thanks the client every time, and the class usually responds by clapping. In the few classes I have sat in on other than Mr. Dana's, the facilitator usually just points and calls on the client then moves on. Mr. Dana's slightly different approaches in all his classes have begun to add up in my mind.

0

Mr. Dana: "Julian, I haven't forgotten you. Please go ahead if you would like."

Julian: "Thanks, Mr. Dana. Natalie and I have the same therapist. I have the same list, so I don't need to read them out as well to the class, do I? I do try to read the list every morning while I'm standing in front of the mirror. Sometimes, I forget to do them. I don't see anything happening when I do them."

Mr. Dana: "No worries, thanks, man. Julian, one reason you're not noticing a difference or getting the full effect of the positive affirmations is you are only *trying* to do them Anything you are being asked to do must be done consistently. All of you did your addiction in a consistent manner with all you had. You never *tried* to go gamble, get a drink, or get high. You did it. *Trying* means *attempting*, not *doing*.

"Look, in the English language there are only twenty-six letters in the alphabet—"

0

Mac: Mr. Dana went to the blackboard and in capital letters wrote the letters "A" and "B."

0

Mr. Dana continued: "Is there a letter that goes between the letter A and the letter B? Of course not. The same goes for trying. In recovery you are either all in or all out. Exactly like the letters A and B. Nothing comes in between those letters. In recovery, you are *doing* recovery or *not doing* recovery. I call it *Donting*. Yeah, I made up a word— *Donting*. You are either doing or not doing. Not doing is called *Donting*. There is no *try* or *trying*. It is either A or B. That's it. 'A' is *doing* and 'B' is *donting*.

"So the question again is, why aren't you willing to put in your best effort and do those affirmations consistently? Of course none of you will see any type of effect if you only do those affirmations—or for that matter, anything in the program—with relentless commitment. Stop trying. *Do!*

"Let's take a look at these two clients' affirmations. What we have seen with these two clients is that they say the exact same things every morning from the same list. Now, I'm not a therapist. As I have said many times, I barely got out of high school. I would never find fault in anyone's approach, especially a therapist who has gone on to a higher level of education. I will never ridicule or be negative about anyone's approach or suggestions if they are done in a positive manner. For me"—Mr. Dana pointed to himself— "listen closely, I'm saying *only me*, I believe the affirmation *must* come from in here"—he pointed to his heart—"and here"—he pointed to his head—"the *real truth!* You are rejoining the heart and mind, which is creating a unity of spirit.

"When anyone is doing a mirror affirmation, they need to feel it, believe it, and mean it. I am not finding criticism in these lists. Shit, no offense to Natalie, Julian, their therapist, or anyone else with those lists. Personally, I don't believe half the stuff on those lists about myself, and if I don't believe them, how can I actually do them? The positivity of the lists are a great start. That's the important part. That should be the affirmation! 'I am starting to say positive things to myself.'"

Mr. Dana walked to the blackboard and wrote the word AFFIRMATION in capital letters.

"The definition of an affirmation is the"—Mr. Dana underlined the letters FIRM twice—"validation, validity, or truth of something. The 'firming' up of a thought or statement. Now, affirmations do not always have to be positive. For instance, 'I am a terrible person, a liar, a cheat, and a lousy parent.' That is telling a negative truth from the past and 'firming' up a thought. It is a negative thought, of course; however, I am affirming the truth of something even though it is a negative affirmation.

"The emphasis needs to be on a continuing, relentless commitment, every day, to say something to ourselves that is positive. Keep in mind that we've all done badly to ourselves and others in our addictions. You must understand that you did not do terrible things every day of your life. I admit I was a shitty, selfish parent, only caring for myself and my addiction. However, when I can look back with clarity, I see that at times I was a good parent. I took my kids to ballet lessons twice a week. I bought them—at times— nice birthday and Christmas presents, etc. etc. If I'm going to confront skeletons from my past, of which there are plenty, I'm going to pull out a few dusty trophies from that past as well. That creates some semblance of balance in my life today. None of us did despicable acts to those we love twenty-four/seven. At times we did okay. That is what you hold on to.

"I was an addict for thirty-five years. I did not ruin anyone's life three hundred and sixty-five days a year for thirty-five years except mine!"

Mr. Dana went on, "What we must understand is that when we use any type of word and speak it out loud, the sound comes out of our mouths and into our ears. When we hear with our ears, it goes into the brain. When we have 'words of thought' or self-talk, these thoughts or self-talk go straight to the brain as well.

"What do we think or self-talk about all day? Be conscious of these things. If I'm talking to myself, I am gonna say good things or say positive affirmations. It's that simple. When we go to bed and lay there alone with our most private thoughts before going to sleep, what are we saying? Anyone? Go ahead, Ms. Cecilia."

Cecilia started to share but was interrupted at times by her slight crying. "All day I walk around thinking I hope my kids don't get taken away by CPS." (Crying.) "I go to sleep and think of my children going to a foster mom." (Crying softly.) "I go to bed worrying about CPS and tell myself what a lousy mother I am." (Crying louder.)

Mr. Dana: "Ms. C., first, thank you for being honest and sharing."

The class clapped lightly.

"I understand how difficult the program has been for you. Keep in mind that you are doing everything you can for yourself and your kids right now. You are not a lousy mom today. So stop thinking those negative affirmations before bed. At bedtime tell yourself you are doing everything you can to resurrect what your addiction took away. Say something like, 'Being in the program is helping me. Helping my children and helping the legal situation I am in.'

"That is not being a lousy mom. Do you know and realize how hard you've been working in this program every single day? I see it, the staff sees it, the clients see it, and most importantly, your CFS worker is being told this. I hope you now start to see this as well. You are helping yourself and your children daily!

"You see, right there is *your* positive affirmation." He looked around the classroom and told them, "The affirmation Ms. C. should be doing at night is, 'I am doing all I can do to help myself. I am doing all I can to help my children every single day.' You don't need a list for that. It

116

comes from here"—he pointed to his heart—"and here"—he pointed to his head.

Mr. Dana continued, "Anyone in here a real cook? Matthew, I heard you're a chef. Is that true?"

From the back of the classroom, Matthew answered shyly, "Yes, I am. I was the head chef at the Hilton Hotel in La Canada, but I was suspended. The HR Department said I have a drinking problem. The Hilton said I was ordering way to much alcohol. They finally figured out I was putting too much wine, champagne, and cognac in me . . . and none in any of the food!"

The class and Mr. Dana cracked up loudly.

Mr. Dana, still laughing and shaking his head a bit, said, "I have a cooking problem. I need your expertise. Would it be alright if I ask you a cooking question?"

Matthew brightened. "Sure. I'd love to help you."

Mr. Dana: "Tonight when I get home, I have a really tough piece of skirt steak. I want it tasty and not tough for tomorrow's dinner. I have people coming over. Should I leave the steak in the refrigerator tonight and, when I get home tomorrow, just throw it on the barbeque?"

Matthew: "Absolutely not. Skirt steak is a really, really tough piece of meat. What I suggest is that when you get home tonight, take it out of the fridge and pour some pineapple juice and soy sauce all over it. Cover it up and put it back in the fridge until about an hour before you barbeque tomorrow. You want the meat to marinate overnight. The marinade will take the toughness out of the meat by seeping into the meat overnight. If you don't have pineapple juice, use a Coke. You need sweetness. The sugar, along with the salt of the soy sauce, will break down the toughness of the meat. And it'll taste good, too."

Mr. Dana: "Thanks, Matt. Maybe you can come over tomorrow night and cook dinner for me?" Mr. Dana waited while the class laughed at his humor and then he continued, "Marinate. Marinate to get the toughness out. Use sweetness and salt for flavor. You heard the chef." He pointed to his head and said, "This piece of meat in my head is called a brain. Every night when I go to sleep worrying, thinking what a shitty parent I am, thinking and being frustrated about something that happened during the day or the past, endlessly endlessly tossing and turning in my sleep, what flavors am I marinating"—again he pointed to his head— "my brain in? If negative thoughts were flavors 'seeping in' overnight, what flavors am I allowing to seep into the meat?" He again pointed to his head. "As addicts, all of our brains are fucking tougher than a skirt steak. These negative affirmations only increase the toughness." He pointed to the blackboard "Remember, I am 'firming' up a thought. I am adding validity to this thought. Would anyone eat a skirt steak if it was marinated in shit and piss all night?"

The class shouted, "No," and booed.

"Of course not. It would taste like shit and piss. What flavors are you marinating your brain in? You see, when you go to bed at night, use positive affirmations. Use some flavoring, add some sweetness. Say things like, 'I stayed in the program one more day. I'm proud that I am clean today. I will give even more to the program tomorrow and invest further in myself.' You don't need a list for these thoughts. What you need is *awareness*.

"Marinate these types of thoughts before bed. Let these words of thought seep into your brain. Make yourself do this through practice, practice, practice. The more you practice, the better you get. That is how to become a champion. Through daily, ongoing practice.

"Look, when class first started, I told all of you to follow the 'thread.' Realize that the thread is always *this* lesson, a *previous* lesson, or the *next* lesson. A simple, long, thin thread.

0

Mac: Mr. Dana took out several long pieces of thread from his bag. He held one thread in one of his hands. In the other hand, he held another long thread. He began showing these threads to the class, lifting them up and down.

0

Mr. Dana continued, "I need you all to really imagine these long, thin pieces of thread as separate tools or lessons. Each thread is a tool or lesson. And see this? It's another piece of thread." He held up another thread. "You all see these long threads?"

The class, in unison, replied, "Yes."

Mr. Dana: "Good. Now, when I start twisting and twisting these long threads, and I mean *really* twisting them together, they make a piece of string."

0

Mac: Mr. Dana began twisting the threads together. He continued to twist those threads over and over and over, actually making me believe he was twisting his classes together with the threads he had in his hands. Then he took out several long pieces of string from his bag.

0

Mr. Dana: "These two pieces of thread have turned into a single strand of string. You all see this piece of string I made with the thread?"

The class again responded in unison with a resounding, "Yes!"

Mr. Dana: "When I twist two pieces of string together, they make twine. See?" He pulled a piece of twine from his bag. "And I keep twisting the threads into string, and twisting the string into twine." He was twisting and twisting with every word. "Then I take the twine and twist it repeatedly, and remember, these threads, strings, and twine are all your prior and future class lessons, along with all your tools you have acquired."

0

Mac: As Mr. Dana kept talking, he never stopped twisting the twine. He would stop and look at it and then twist some more.

0

Mr. Dana, excited now: "You all see? The twine has turned into rope!" He held up a piece of rope he had taken from the bag. "Look. From thread to string to twine to rope. This rope each of you make is for you to climb out of the fucking hole you put yourself in!

"If you don't twist each piece together every day, every damn day . . . good luck climbing out of your hole with you only holding a piece of thread. It ain't gonna happen.

"I hope you all remember that a while back I told all of you there would be a test on foundational tools. Can anyone here tell me all six?"

Someone in the class shouted, "Faith in yourself."

Another one shouted, "Mental Discipline."

Mr. Dana: "Hold up. Hold up. Don't shout one or two. Someone raise their hand if they know all six."

Charlene raised her hand and said, "I got it right here in my notes, Mr. Dana." Charlene looked frantically through her notebook.

Mr. Dana ran to Charlene and said loudly, passionately, "Every one of you who does not know these foundational tools through daily practice is wasting your time here in the program. None of you are going to be walking around after the program with these notes"—he grabbed Charlene's notebook and waved it over his head— "in your hand. Situations will come up and what are you going to say, 'Excuse me, let me get my notes from my addictive recovery program?' You have either practiced them for ninety days in the program or not.

"I made you all a bet at the start of this program about practicing these tools daily. It looks like no one is going to win the bet. It seems my reputation and ID are safe at this point. But, for all of you, there is still time to win."

0

Mac: Mr. Dana was referring to the bet he made the first day of his class. He bet his students that if, after using the foundational tools for the ninety days of the program and for thirty days afterwards, they found that the foundational tools didn't work, he would give up his reputation and his ID.

0

Mr. Dana: "The foundational tools need to be instilled in your head and heart. Instinctual! Instinctual means actions without thought. Most of you know who Kobe Bryant is, of course. Kobe won five NBA championships, eighteen times he was an All-Star MVP, he led the league in scoring twice. When Kobe was asked how he got so good at shooting from anywhere on the floor, he said, 'I practice at home every day. I shoot over two thousand shots from all angles. The shooting becomes instinctual. When the game is on the line, I don't *think*, I *shoot*. I practice, practice, and practice. That's how I stay a champion.'

"You hear what Kobe said? When the game is on the line, when your *lives* are on the line, you better practice, practice, practice. These foundational tools *must* be instinctual. Action without thought.

"Nothing will free you. Not unless you start now and use what is being offered. All day, every day. Revolution. I am giving you a piece of thread right now. For some of you, realize it is your last fucking move. Why aren't you making it your best move?

"The problem as I see it is that a majority in here look at recovery as a jail sentence, a big hassle, or a toothache. Change your mindset. It is a beautiful thing to reignite your Spirit and be who God meant you to be. You all need to be singing all day long and know God will love you all day long if you let Him! You need *enthusiasm* for this program."

0

Mac: Mr. Dana went to the blackboard and wrote "Enthusiasm" in large letters. He then underlined the first five letters of the word.

0

Mr. Dana: "'Enthu' in Latin is 'En Theo.' That means 'in God.' Inspired by God. Passion. You need to be inspired by God by having enthusiasm! It is the only way. Each and every day. Enthusiasm.

0

Mac: Mr. Dana was making an emphatic plea with the clients to use this time to change by utilizing what was being offered in the program.

0

Mr. Dana: "You must use your foundational tools all day. They are affirmations. Say to yourself all day, 'I believe in myself, I have faith in myself, I do not doubt myself today. I have mental discipline to do these things daily. I have self-motivation, as the results are an investment in me, and I have relentless commitment. I cannot be stopped.'

"These are affirmations to do not only at night before bed. You need to do them all during the day as well. Stop *trying* . . . you must *do*. Marinate yourself with these thoughts all day and all night. Pay attention to your internal voice. What is that voice saying all day? It is your voice and your choice."

0

Mac: Mr. Dana then went into his bag and pulled out a normal, empty, ten-ounce water glass. He set it on the podium. Then he pulled out a ziplock baggie filled with what looked like sand.

0

Mr. Dana said to the class, "See this clear, empty glass? This glass represents my life. Do you all see this baggie filled with sand? This sand represents all my problems. It represents my tax issues with the damn IRS. The lien on my weekly check from unpaid bills accrued during my addiction. It represents the problems my addiction has caused with my children. This sand represents my pain from losing a very close family member recently. In other words, imagine this sand as every issue or problem I have or you have. Now watch as I pour all this sand into this glass. Please remember that this sand represents my life. See how it all fits nicely in the glass? I would say this glass is about three-quarters full of sand."

0

Mac: Mr. Dana put the empty ziplock bag back into the bag. He then pulled out three golf balls.

0

Mr. Dana continued, "You see these three golf balls? Look at how I wrote the first three foundational tools, one tool on each ball."

0

Mac: Mr. Dana held up the first golf ball and written on it was the word "Believe." He then put the first golf ball into the glass of sand.

0

Mr. Dana: "You see this first golf ball that says 'Believe?' See how easily it fits with all my problems?"
A few in the class yelled, "Yes."

0

Mac: Mr. Dana held up the second golf ball, which was labeled "Faith." He put it into the glass on top of the first golf ball.

124

0

Mr. Dana: "Now, I take this second golf ball marked 'Faith' and put it right on top of the first golf ball. I 'Believe' and have 'Faith' in all my issues. You all see?"

Again, the class responded with, "Yes."

0

Mac: Mr. Dana then took the third golf ball, which was marked "No Doubts." He tried to put it into the glass on top of the other golf balls, except that third golf ball wouldn't fit and fell to the floor.

Mr. Dana tried again with the same result. The golf ball wouldn't fit, and it kept falling out of the glass. It seemed that Mr. Dana was getting irritated. I thought he hadn't measured correctly with the sand and now was realizing he had made a mistake.

0

Mr. Dana: "Fuck. These three golf ball tools don't fit in the glass with all my issues, the sand."

Some in the class laughed.

"Hmmm. Maybe I have too many issues. Okay, how about this?"

0

Mac: Out of his bag, Mr. Dana took another empty glass exactly like the first one. He took the two golf balls out of the glass with the sand and put them into the empty glass. He then took the third golf ball and put it into the glass on top of the other two golf balls.

0

Mr. Dana: "With this empty glass, I have plenty of room for all three golf balls. Look, can you all see that the three golf balls fit into the glass without any sand? Then, I take this first glass holding the sand, and I pour it on top of the three golf balls. You see? Do you see how the sand—my issues—goes under and between the three golf balls—the foundational tools—and fills the crevices? All the sand fits into the glass—which is my life—just fine."

0

Mac: Mr. Dana went into his bag and pulled out another ziplock baggie filled with more sand. He showed it to the class.

0

Mr. Dana: "You see, by putting my three foundational tools first—which is really putting *me* first before my issues—they fit perfectly in my life. I need to always come before anything. Before my children, work, family, whatever. I need to always do *me* first. You need to do *you* first, and your children, work, and issues will fit all around you like the sand in the glass."

0

Mac: Mr. Dana took the second baggie with the additional sand and started to pour.

0

126

Mr. Dana continued, "You see this second baggie of sand? Those are all *your* problems. When I do *me* first, I have room for all of *my* problems and all of *yours* as well."

0

Mac: Mr. Dana poured the second bag of sand on top of his three golf balls and the original sand. The second bag of sand fit as well.

0

Mr. Dana: "I have to take care of myself first, always put myself first. Then I have ample room for my problems and all of your problems. Do you see how all the sand—our issues—fits in the glass—my life—just fine?"

The class clapped enthusiastically.

Mr. Dana: "Each of us has only one job on earth to do. Only one. That job is to do *You*. Do *You* the best you can. I do my only job, which is *Me*, the best I can. By doing *Me* first the best I can, it makes me a better father, husband, teacher, friend, person.

"*Do Your Job*. A lot of you are here for the simple reason that you didn't do your job well enough. Ms. Cecilia is probably a good mom at times, even when she was loaded. Mr. Matthew is probably a pretty good chef, even when drinking the cooking wine."

The class laughed.

"But Cecilia will be a better mother when she does her *only* job . . . which is to do *her* first. Matthew will be a better chef when he does his job first, which is *taking care of himself*. Taking care of self in a beautiful way is your only job on earth. Taking care of yourself in a spiritual, mental, and physical way. You are creating perfect harmony and balance in your life. That is God's plan.

"I told you earlier that God is always giving us hints and clues if we are tuned in to hearing and seeing His message. Today, there is a fire burning out of control in Australia. There is a terrible drought in India. You all might have read about the huge, seven-point-four earthquake in Columbia or the tsunami in Fiji. These natural occurrences happen every day on earth. Every day.

"When an earthquake hits the Earth, does the Earth stop? Does the Earth yell out to the Sun and say, 'I am not going to rotate today and go around you anymore?'"

The class laughed.

"Fuck no! The Earth still does its job. It rotates around the Sun—six hundred and seven million miles a year at seventy-seven thousand and six miles per hour—regardless of what is going on. The Earth does its job. Learn from this! God is giving you a hint.

"And when your life has tsunamis, hurricanes, and drought—I call them life-quakes—do you run? Do you stop? Fuck no! Be like the Earth and keep going. None of you have a monopoly on life-quakes. We all have them. Learn to get better at handling these life-quakes. Do your job.

"Anyone in here have a particularly good idea what would happen if our Sun just stopped? I mean, the Sun suddenly stopped doing its job, simply shut off. Give me a couple examples of how it would effect Earth. Anyone?"

Dre raised his hand and said, "Well, it would go dark on earth and get cold."

"Mr. Dana: "That is correct. It would not only get dark, it would get black and freezing. How about the planets in the solar system? Go ahead, Ms. Lolli."

Ms. Lolli: "I think the Sun keeps the planets in alignment or something like that."

Mr. Dana: "Absolutely. This enables the planets to

orbit the Sun due to the Sun's gravity. Okay, now what happens to the planets if the Sun doesn't do its job? Go ahead, Ms. Bonnie."

Ms. Bonnie: "The planets would float away?"

Mr. Dana: "Exactly. If nothing is holding the planets in place, they would float away or crash into each other. That is what would happen if the Sun did not do its job every day.

"When all of you did not do your job, the 'planets' in your orbit floated away. Your spouse floated out of your life, your kids, your employment, your friends, money, health, emotions all crashed into each other or floated out of your orbit. You did not do your job. And if you do your only job, which is *You*, these things will be attracted back. Doing your job will create energy, bringing these things back into your orbit. Do your *only* job, which is YOU! God gives us hints and clues. Study the universe."

0

Mac: Mr. Dana paced around the podium, firing the "real truth" on all cylinders and in all directions. He was a man possessed, a whirling dervish. The clients were entranced. Class had already run twenty-five minutes longer than scheduled, which was cutting into the clients' rec time. But no one moved or said a word. No one wanted to break the vibe, the energy, the "spell" we were all under and witnessing.

0

Mr. Dana: "I hear all the time, 'I want recovery for my kids, my spouse, whatever, etc. etc.' All of you had these things in your life and you still got fucking high. Stop saying you are here in recovery for someone or something else. You are

129

here in recovery to learn to do *your one job,* which is *You.* What you did *not* do was your job. That is why you are here now. To learn how to *do your fucking job!*"

The class cheered.

Mr. Dana: "Ok, one final demonstration today. Oh shit! Class is way over into your rec time. We can do it next time, if I remember."

The class yelled out a chorus of, "NO, NO, please go on, Mr. Dana. Please, please."

Mr. Dana, laughing: "Really? Okay, if you all insist. Anyone who wants to go to rec time, go now. I'm serious. Anyone can go. Really? None of you want to leave class? Wow. Today, I am so grateful to all of you. I truly am. You humble me." He looked toward the heavens and said, "Thank you, God.

0

Mac: No one got up. I truly sat in amazement. The clients were choosing to stay. I had never seen this before. Then Mr. Dana went into his "magic bag of tricks" again and took out what looked like a small, inexpensive mirror.

0

Mr. Dana: "Relax, all of you. This little, pink mirror is from The Dollar Tree. It's just a two-dollar mirror, so don't start getting all nervous. In this last demonstration, all of you will do the demonstrating. All of you, pay attention to everyone's body language and be serious, please. No fucking around. And remember, none of you ever have to participate in any of my classes. If you don't want to participate, simply pass the mirror."

0

Dana Axelrod

Mac: Mr. Dana handed the mirror to the first client, a man named Trent.

0

Mr. Dana: "This exercise is really quite easy. Look in the mirror and ask yourself out loud, 'Who am I?' Simply look into the mirror and say two or three things about yourself. Then pass the mirror to the person next to you. And be fucking serious, no games or laughing. We're all sharing in here. Even Mac can have a go at it!"

The class laughed.

0

Mac: Mr. Dana knows I'm only here to take notes and observe in his classes. In addition, the clients can revoke this privilege. I do my best to sit unnoticed and not take away from the bond between students and teacher.

0

Trent, holding the mirror: "I am a grateful, a kinder, recovering drug addict." He passed the mirror to the client sitting next to him.

0

Mac: I noticed a few clients seemed to be uneasy with this exercise. Marcos had the mirror now.

0

Marcos: "I'm a strong, extremely handsome man"—the class laughed—"and I am also a terrible person. I have done

131

so much dirt and damage. I really hate myself for what I did to my wife and kids."

The class clapped as Marcos passed the mirror and looked at Mr. Dana.

Mr. Dana: "Remember, when you ask, 'Who am I?' say it to the mirror, not me or anyone else. It's important that you look yourself in the eye and tell yourself who you are."

Juliette, stuttering: "I-I am . . . I really don't want to do this." She quickly passed the mirror.

0

Mac: The mirror was passed client to client. Some clients were willing to confront who they were; some were honest, some passed the mirror.

0

Mr. Dana admonished a few clients by saying, "I see you people all day talking outside. All day. Talking in classes when you shouldn't, and now, when it gets serious, you can't even open your mouth and say something about yourself? You all better *know* who you are. Begin to *be* that person before leaving this facility. It's only a two-dollar mirror."

Kyra, after a long stare in the mirror, said in a confident voice, "I am Kyra. I am in recovery and proud of that today. I do *believe* in myself today. I have *faith* in myself and in a *Higher Power*. I do not *doubt* myself. I want recovery to learn to be a better person to myself. I want to learn to do my only job on earth the best I can. When I do my job better, I will be a better person to my children, my husband, my friends. As Mr. Dana always says, the number one affirmation has to be—"

0

Mac: Kyra looked into the mirror and yelled the same thing three or four times, very loudly.

0

"—Why Not Me? Why NOT Me? WHY NOT ME?"

The class went bonkers with approval. Someone in the class called out to Mr. Dana, "Look into the mirror, Mr. Dana. Who are you?"

Several others called, "Yeah, Mr. Dana, who are you?"

Mr. Dana looked into the mirror then put it back into the bag and in a loud, firm, unwavering, voice, stated, "You think I need a mirror to know who I am? I am Dana Fucking Axelrod. Do you all not see who I am? You all are *my* mirror." He gestured to the entire class. "The way each person, client, stranger, or staff member talks to me or treats me is a reflection of me. I *know* who I am. I am *being*, all day, *who* I am. I don't need no stinking mirror."

The class laughed.

Mr. Dana: "Class, join me in saying the number one affirmation, which after time will pay dividends in self-confidence, self-esteem, and self-worth. Let's say this affirmation together. 'Why Not Me?'"

The class repeated, "Why not me?"

Mr. Dana: "Louder. 'Why Not Me?'"

Together, the class and Mr. Dana yelled, "Why Not Me?"

Mr. Dana: "Again."

The class in unison screamed, "Why Not Me. Why Not Me?"

Quietly now, Mr. Dana said, "Thank you, class. I don't know why not you. You all are as good or better than anyone out there. Once you *know* who you are, *be* who you are, *believe* in who you are, have *faith* in who you are, and stop *doubting* who you are, when you put all five together, you will shine like the Sun. Then, instead of asking, 'Why not me?' all of you will be able to smile in the mirror and say, 'IT IS ME!' Class dismissed."

The clients walked out the door, cheering and chanting, "Why Not Me?"

Smart Versus Strong

Mac: Of course, Mr. Dana came walking in on time and appeared to be in a lighthearted mood. On the way to the podium he stopped to talk with several clients. I could not hear what was being said, but the group he was talking to broke up laughing. Mr. Dana was laughing as he approached the podium.

0

Mr. Dana: "Well, well, well. If it isn't some of the greatest people 'hungry' for recovery. I, Mr. Dana, am here to satisfy your hunger, and I plan on feeding all of you a fantastic meal. My hope is that it will only increase your desire for more of this precious food I'm serving.

"I look around at this entire class. Man, some of you men are fierce looking. If I was a stranger and any of you came walking down the street, I would cross the street. You all look so big and scary. Shit, you men are some of the toughest I've seen in a group."

The class laughed.

0

Mac: I didn't know where this is going, but I have learned to expect the unexpected from Mr. Dana, both in his approach and his teaching style. Along with the other clients, I'm waiting to see where Mr. Dana is leading us. Call it suppressed excitement.

0

Mr. Dana: "Do all of you men work out every chance you get? You all look so strong. Looking at all you men, I see a tough, strong, collective group. I know a majority of you have also done some 'time.' Strong and tough, that's what you all are. No doubt about that."

0

Mac: Now Mr. Dana turned his attention to all the ladies in the classroom.

0

Mr. Dana: "Don't worry, ladies, you're tougher and stronger than the men. Also prettier!"

The class laughed and the men made assorted booing noises, all in good-natured fun.

0

Mac: I saw another facet to Mr. Dana's teachings. He was having fun, joking a bit, and had dialed down his passion. A true maestro.

0

Mr. Dana: "I'm going to tell you why the ladies in here are tougher and stronger. First off, during their addiction, they have been through everything you men have been through. It was most likely a lot harder for them. In addition, most of these"—he gestured around the classroom—"ladies have done some time, as well. But they are stronger than you men due to the fact that they have the ability to bring new life into this world. You men, think how strong these ladies have to be. Carrying a baby human being in their stomachs for nine months . . . now *that* is tough and strong.

"However, that's not the only reason why they're stronger. The *real* reason they're so tough is that they used to put up with us." He pointed to himself and around the classroom. "That's right. What made ladies so damn tough is that at one time or another, they put up with us men!"

The ladies in the classroom cheered and clapped; the men booed.

Mr. Dana: "Ok, ok, let's not get carried away. Settle down. Unfortunately, whether you're male or female and the strongest person on the planet, it won't help your overcome your addictions. Look, I think back to my addictive days . . . going days without sleep, going to work twelve to fourteen hours a day. Getting knocked down by my addiction every fucking day and getting up for more. I was fucking tough and strong.

"I know all of you are just as strong or stronger than I was. As I have said before, addicts are the strongest motherfuckers on planet Earth. My god, the things we survive. They should make a TV show called *The Addicts' Survival Island*, showcasing how nothing can stop us. Match us addicts against those *Survival Island* contestants every Sunday night on CBS."

Mr. Dana and the class cracked up. It was obvious that everyone thought the idea was hilarious.

Mr. Dana: "No, seriously, being tough and strong is not the way to beat any addiction. You've all heard those phrases like, 'Be Strong,' 'Stay Strong,' blah, blah, blah. Don't believe that crap. Recovery is not about being strong. The only way to beat any addiction is by being fucking *smart*!

"Men, you better start getting smart. The women have already smartened up and are no longer allowing or putting up with our shit. I telling you men the *real truth*. Anyway, yeah, I said, being strong won't work in recovery.

I don't care how strong you are; the world is full of tough, strong men and women. Have you ever asked yourselves why some of these tough three-hundred-pound men working in some smelt mine in Bulgaria or on the Siberian railroad aren't the heavyweight champ? The world is filled with big, tough, strong men and women. Why aren't they world champions? I'll tell you why. Boxing is called the 'sweet science.' That term is applied to the smart boxer. It comes down to a boxer in front of thousands of fans and millions more on Pay TV to win by being smart. The smart boxer is able to calculate, strategize, and develop a plan during the fight. Using his brain to instantly read the opponent and come up with a winning formula.

"You can sit there and say to yourself, 'Bullshit, we're talking about addiction not boxing.' You would most definitely be wrong. I am going to hammer away at your old ways of thinking by repeating new tools for you to employ over and over. The reason why I repeat everything is so you keep getting this new knowledge etched into your brains. New facts and a new way to look at recovery. Again, etched in your brains. Repetition.

"Think how many times you repeated the same thing over and over in your addiction. I have already proven to all of you how good you all got by practicing your addiction daily. Practicing over and over new thoughts every day will be the new way to act in recovery. Look, you don't have to believe me. I can prove to all of you that smart always wins out over strong.

"I'm going to give you a couple of examples. Let's look back into history, shall we? The Trojan War as reported by Homer in the *Iliad*. It was the Greeks against the city of Troy. The strongest, toughest, Greek fighters to ever assemble surrounded the city of Troy. I mean, the Greeks had Ulysses! I hope some of you know who he was. They had Atlas, that's the guy who holds up the world! You think he was strong? He holds up the fucking Earth! His strength didn't matter against the walls of Troy.

"You see, the big problem was that the Greeks could not bring down the strong walls surrounding Troy. No matter how hard they tried. So what did the Greeks do after ten years of war?" Mr. Dana pointed to his head and continued, "Ulysses used his brain because he realized that being strong didn't work. Smart versus strong. Ulysses used his brain and came up with a plan to build this big wooden horse and leave it at the massive gates of Troy as a gift. Then Ulysses used his smart skills again and had all the Greek ships leave. We're talking over a thousand ships. The battlefield was deserted.

"The Trojans saw that gift the Greeks had left. The Trojans brought this 'gift horse' inside their protective, strong walls. There was one small problem, though. Ulysses and a small band of warriors had hidden inside this gift' horse. After the Trojans had partied and fell asleep, Ulysses and his SWAT team climbed out of this huge, gift horse and killed them all.

"Being strong didn't work against the strength of the Trojan army and their walls. What won the Trojan War was Ulysses using his mind, his brain, his *smarts*!

"You're all strong. I already told all of you how tough and strong you all are. Strong will *not* work against the strength of addiction. It won't stand up and beat the strength of addiction. To win this war, you need to be fucking smart. This is a perfect example of *smart* versus *strong*."

Mr. Dana continued, "Any of you know about malware, encryption, and anti-virus measures in computers?"

Ernesto raised his hand and spoke. "Yeah, it's to

secure data and prevent hacking. Malware is the attacking virus."

Mr. Dana: "Exactly. They call that 'worm' or malware a Trojan horse. Why? It's because that 'attacking virus' is so smart. The Trojan horse! Another example of smart versus strong.

"For those of you who do not believe in Greek History or Homer's *Iliad*, perhaps some of you are religious and would like another example of smart versus strong. I'm gonna make this quick. In the Old Testament, in First Samuel, Chapter Seventeen, there's a story about a giant of a man approximately seven feet tall. This giant was a killer. A philistine. Nobody could stand up to this massive killer. He was big, strong, and massive, exactly like the wall surrounding Troy.

"Now this giant wanted to fight any man among the Hebrews. No one wanted to die, no one wanted to fight this giant, except for one man—or should I say one *young* man. This young man was a fifteen- year-old shepherd named David. David volunteered to fight the giant. The giant's name was Goliath. David and Goliath. Most of you know the story.

"You see, David knew that if he came close to Goliath, he would be killed exactly like all the other fighters before him. What did David do? David used his fucking brain, that's what he did. He found a couple of rocks, put them in his slingshot, and hit Goliath right in the forehead from twenty-five feet away. Goliath fell down dead. David then went up to Goliath and cut the big dummy's head off! Only when Goliath was dead did David approach him. David was *smart* enough to know *not* to go against someone stronger than himself. He was *smart* enough to know to cut Goliath's head off after he was dead . . . not *before*. He used his fucking head.

"All of you, use your heads, not your strength. Your strength won't work against the strength of the 'dark side.' God gave you a brain to counter strength.

"Now, I have one more example of smart versus strong. Some of you know and can attest to this true, modern-day story. If you don't want to learn from ancient texts, learn from modern-day facts. Don't be resistant to what I'm saying. That's your addiction rebelling. I ask right now for you to open your minds to what I am attempting to illustrate to you. To teach you.

"In 1974 there was a giant of a man. He was twenty-five years old and the heavyweight champion of the world. His name was George Foreman. Foreman's record at that time was forty to zero, with thirty-seven of those wins coming by knockout. Now, that's a strong punch. Thirty-seven knockouts against grown men. Foreman was *strong*. My God, Foreman was a beast.

"Then came his fight against Mohammad Ali. Ali was thirty-two years old and, at that point in his career, wasn't much of a knockout fighter. In Ali's past fights he would run and dance around the ring. That wasn't going to work against Foreman. What was Ali gonna do? Ali used his brain. What Ali did was lay way back—and I mean way, way, way back—against the ropes and let Foreman punch his body for seven rounds. Foreman punched Ali's body non-stop for seven rounds! The thing was, Ali knew that, with the heat—" Mr. Dana paused and asked, "Did I tell you the fight was in Africa and the temperature was over a hundred degrees?"

The class, enthralled, yelled out, "No."

Mr. Dana continued his story: "Ali knew from the heat and the way Foreman was punching away that Foreman was getting tired. Ali said after the fight, 'By the fifth round, his punches were so slow, and they did not have any effect whatsoever on my body.'

"Even though everyone in attendance, including the fight announcers, all reported that Foreman was killing Ali by 'punishing' Ali's body, Ali knew different. He used his brain, the 'sweet science.' Ali knocked Foreman out in the eighth round. The name of the tactic used by Ali is the 'Rope a Dope.' Think about it. Rope a *dope*. That is another great example of smart versus strong. Ali used his *smarts* against a strong *dope*.

"The thing is, no one thought Ali could win that fight. No one in the sporting world. The so called 'experts' thought Foreman was too big, too strong. Ali was the underdog. The odds were five to one. No one thought Ali had a chance. Do any of you know how big the payoff is on an underdog? It's huge.

"Smart versus strong."

0

Mac: Mr. Dana went from a voice of cheerful entertainment to one of deep seriousness. The class was suddenly quiet . . . still. I could feel the change of energy, and I observed the faces of the clients who were listening intently. The clients always *paid rapt attention when Mr. Dana spoke from the heart.*

0

Mr. Dana continued in an intense manner, "All of you in here right now are underdogs. No one expects you to win this fight, this battle, this war. Most people are betting against you. The payoff of an underdog is huge. When—not *if*— *when* you win this war against addiction, the payoff for each of you is *huge*.

"Notice that I'm using the word 'when' not 'if.' I am using my tool of words. Repetition and tools together. Use all the tools you are learning, all the time and all together. Don't *try*. *Do*! Use those who doubt you for inspiration. Use the underdog role for motivation. Feed off those things to go forward with your life."

0

Mac: Mr. Dana handed out to all the clients pictures of the inside of the world's largest libraries. He then went and taped a few of those pictures to the blackboard.

0

Mr. Dana: "I want all of you to look at these pictures. There are millions of books on these shelves." He motioned to the pictures on the blackboard and continued, "This particular picture is the Library of Congress. This one is a photo of their law library. All of these books of law you see in this picture total approximately two-point-nine-million books. There are forty million books in this one library alone." Again, he pointed to the pictures on the blackboard.

"That's a lot of books. I want you all to look at any one of the pictures I have given you of the world's biggest libraries. Now, holding any picture you choose, I want you to imagine that, out of all these millions of books, there is also a librarian at your library. Really imagine that you are at one of these libraries. You hear the librarian tell you—"

Mr. Dana began imitating an elderly woman's voice. "You can read *any* book in this library except for two books." Now, each of take a pen, a pencil, a crayon, whatever and do this—"

0

Mac: Mr. Dana went to the photo of the Library of Congress with its millions of books and, taking a red marker, and put a large X on two books.

0

Mr. Dana continued: "With your pen or whatever you have, do what I am doing. Cross off two books out of all the books in the picture you're holding. Everyone do that?"

The class all said, "Yes."

"Now, the librarian in your picture says—" Again, Mr. Dana imitated an elderly woman's voice. "I forgot to tell you, you can read *any* of these books *except* for the two books you crossed out. The titles of the two books you crossed off are *Running Away* and *My Addiction*."

Forcefully, Mr. Dana continued, "Out of all these books, you are never allowed to read the two crossed-off books. Never, never, *never*! To be *smart* you must read all the books you have never read before. If—and I say *if*— you re-read the books *Running Away* and *My Addiction,* that would not be smart at all. You have already read them your whole life. You have re-read those two books over and over and you *know* the endings—they never change—you die!. Read something new. That is how you get smart and stay smart. This library each of you possesses, this library is here"—he pointed to his head—"it contains billions of books full of knowledge. This library is written by *you* and your imagination. This library holds your dreams, desires, hopes.

"All of you know I have sat in the seats you are now sitting in. Some of your counselors here have sat in those seats as well." Mr. Dana pointed to Mac and continued, "Mr. Mac was my client and sat in those exact same seats and heard the exact same things. Mac got smart. Now Mac is highly regarded, highly respected, and highly paid.

"Look, when all of you leave here, you're going to get to the gate. Remember to do this when you leave. I want you to turn around and look at this entire facility. Ask yourself one quick question, 'Did I give my all to change my life while I was here?' You will have your answer instantly. It better be 'Fuck yeah!' Keep in mind that the streets are now brand new and there is nothing you cannot do.

"There are going to be times when you get out of here when you will struggle. That's okay. The struggle is real. But it does get easier through repetition and practice. Show me a person who has stayed clean for ninety days and I will show you a person with courage. Show me a person with six months clean and I will show you a smart fighter.

"I rarely talk much about myself. However, I am going to share a little bit about myself today. I remember going to my very first AA meeting and hearing someone say, 'I haven't had a drink in thirty days.' I was in disbelief. How does someone go thirty days without a drink? I mean, drinking was in my upbringing, in my genes. I started drinking every single day when I was fifteen years old. Every day!

"My dad used to say, 'A man knows the difference between getting fucked up and fucking up.'"

The class laughed.

"What a crock of shit that saying was. Anyway, at the same AA meeting, the next person came up to speak and said, 'I haven't had a drink in two years.' I was floored. I mean *floored*. I remember thinking, *Two years without a drink? No fucking way*! Well, I haven't had a drink or a drug in over eleven years—"

Mr. Dana had to pause while the class clapped wholeheartedly. Then he continued. "Thank you. The point is that my life is so much richer and full today. Do I crave a drink? On a hot day a beer sounds nice. Is a beer going to get me to buy a thousand dollars of meth or coke? Fuck no. I use my tools, though. As I said before, I might *want* a beer, but do I *need* one? Wants versus needs. Smart versus strong. Use your tools together. Repeat them. Practice them.

"I'm going to give you another 'smart' tool. This tool's name is 'Know What Not to Do.' Don't re-read those two books. You know *not* to do that. There will be times when you're sitting at home and a so-called 'friend' asks you to go to the bar, the casino, the G Spot.

The class laughed at that.

"You may think, 'I'm strong, I can go.' What's the Big Book say? 'If you hang around the barber shop, you're going to get a haircut.' That's *not* smart. All these tools or weapons work. Look at Mac, at me, or the other underdogs and know that none of us are better than any of you.

"I have heard and been told that addiction is 'a disease of the brain.' Okay then. If it's a brain disease, and I control my brain, then I am able to control and cure my disease. I am in control of my brain. Doctors can cure some types of cancer, leukemia, Hep, HIV, etc. with a new assortment of medical procedures and drugs. I am telling all of you how to cure your 'brain disease.' Use these new lessons and tools. Smart versus strong. Smart always wins out when facing the strength of addiction. I always repeat everything so you can eat and breathe all I give you all the time. These tools are what you have been hungry for.

"When you are strong and you keep working out, you get stronger. Your muscles get bigger, more toned. People look at you and say, 'Wow, you're getting big, your arms are huge,' whatever. We like that when we work out. We like extrinsic compliments, we like being noticed for hard, disciplined work. Note I said *discipline*. That's a tool, by the way. Now when we work out our brains, no one says, 'Wow, you have a big head.'"

The class laughed.

"No one says, 'Look how strong you are.' When you work out your mind, you get smarter! That's right—your brain gets *smarter*. People will notice and say things like, 'How the fuck did he get so smart?' Or, 'She's so smart,' People will notice, and you can say to yourself, 'I have my own library.'" Mr. Dana pointed to his head. "You will begin to notice that, by doing the smart thing, you are not a 'Rope A Dope' going down for the count like Foreman. You will notice you are winning, like Ali, the underdog. My, what a payoff it is. Huge!

"I am humbled and you are all dismissed. Class over."

Role Models

Mac: Mr. Dana came into class with his speaker on his iPhone blasting a podcast. I believe it was the quarterback Tom Brady's "Let's Go" or "Leading From the Heart." Mr. Dana stood at the podium, putting his fingers to his lips to keep the class quiet and still. Everyone could hear the podcast, and Mr. Dana stood still with his eyes shut for about a minute or so. All we could hear was a voice from the iPhone saying, "—and only with the heart." Mr. Dana put his phone down and shut it off.

0

Mr. Dana: "I love that guy. I mean *love* that guy. Hi, all of you. I am Mr. Dana . . . and you are not!"

The class laughed and Mr. Dana continued, "As usual, I have new knowledge for you. Soak it up, don't dismiss these things I'm going to talk about. You owe it to your soul, to your life, to 'eat the fruits of my wisdom' to grow your spirit. I have told all of you over and over how your addiction has robbed your spirit of light, your life, and your growth. I want all of you to exercise your brain today and get *smarter*, as discussed in the last class. Yes, I am a broken record of recovery and these instruments"—he pointed to his heart and then his head—"only play the same 'greatest hits.' How many of you have a role model, guru, or mentor in your life? Let me see a show of hands please. Okay. A few of you . . . that's good. How many of you know what a role model is? Raise your hands please.

"Hmmm. You three with your hands up, could you share who your role models are? Go ahead, Julian, tell us all who your role model is and why."

Julian: "My grandpa is my role model. The reason why is that he went to work every day for thirty-five years as a barber from Spain. He raised my mother, along with her two sisters and three brothers. He made sure each of his kids and my grandma always had food on the table, a roof over their heads, and he saw to it that all his children graduated high school.

"I remember one thing before he died. I remember playing in the backyard as a kid. One time my grandpa came limping into the garage after work. He did not see me, and he had his hands in an ice bucket and was crying. I . . . never forgot that. He . . . never complained. He . . . never let anyone know the amount of pain he was in. Mr. Dana, he did what . . . you aways say, he did . . . his job. I remember when I was young and once my father yelled at me and said, 'Never let your grandpa hear you complain about that.' Now I know why."

0

Mac: Julian is six-foot-two, weighs about 220 pounds, and has the word "Cholo" tattooed on his neck. Julian almost never shared in class. Now he was sobbing.

0

Mr. Dana: "Julian, thank you so much. I appreciate you opening up. Can I ask you a simple question?"

Julian, "Yeah, I'm cool."

Mr. Dana: "Could you label your grandfather's character or a few of his qualities for us?"

0

Mac: Mr. Dana went to blackboard and wrote as Julian listed his grandfather's qualities.

0

Julian: "A real man. Responsible, never complained."

Mr. Dana continued after turning around from blackboard: "Alright, we have Real, Never Complains, and Responsible. Anyone else have a role model? Go on, Ms. Sabrina, share."

Sabrina: "I got to say my mom. She provided for me and my two little brothers when my dad left us. Worked two, sometimes, three jobs. She taught all of us right and wrong. Always punished us when we did something bad or wrong. I remember getting caught as a teenager for stealing and my mom smacked the shit out of me—"

The entire class laughed at that a lot.

Sabrina continued: "Can I say that? Sorry, Mr. Dana. Anyways, I'm the only one who messed up. My brothers are cool. One is a Marine recruiter and the other works as an EMT driver. I suppose 'hard working,' and 'disciplined morally' would be her character traits."

Mr. Dana wrote that on blackboard then said, "Thanks, Sabrina. It's good to hear you sharing. Okay, we have Hard Working, and Disciplined Morals to add to this list. Anyone else want to share? Yeah, go ahead, Anton."

Anton: "Well, my older brother. He raised all of us after my dad got busted. I was fifteen, my sister was fourteen, and my older brother was, like, nineteen when dad went away. My brother did what he had to do to keep us all together. Took care of business, ya know? I'd say he was a provider."

Mr. Dana wrote PROVIDER on the blackboard and

said, "Thank you, all. So, looking at this list, we see these positive traits up here. All of us can see a pattern. A role model is someone who has a certain pattern or set of behaviors that someone can look up to and want to mirror or model those behaviors. Not all role models are positive, though. A lot of us have had some negative role models we wanted to mirror or model ourselves after. I know some of you wanted to be the next Scarface."

The class laughed.

"Or the next Bonny and Clyde."

More laughter from the class.

"Now, what is important is that you don't have to personally know your role model. Some of you who were wannabe gangsters didn't know Tony Montana in *Scarface*. Yet you wanted to act like him. A majority of you may never wind up achieving the success your role model has achieved. That's okay. You can still act like and have the behaviors of your role model. Remember what I said earlier: 'a certain pattern or behavior to mirror,' That means 'reflect.' We use role models to inspire us. Inspire and to be like. Now take a look at this board behind me and what I wrote. We want to be Real, No Complaints, Responsible, Hard Working, Morally Disciplined, and a Provider.

"I personally have two role models. The first one is the football player Tom Brady."

A few in class booed and yelled, "Cheater." A few cheered.

Mr. Dana: "Knock that shit off. Stop being a hater. None of you know anything about him being a so-called cheater or the facts surrounding 'Deflate Gate.' Even if he did cheat—and he most certainly *did not*—I won't even waste my time or the class's time explaining the real truth to you who booed him and called him a cheat."

He glared at the class and continued, "As I was

saying, even if he did cheat, he still played in ten Super Bowls and has won seven rings! My God, don't boo excellence. You need to learn to revere excellence."

0

Mac: Mr. Dana fiercely defended his role model. I had seen him stand up for the clients this way as well when another staff member wanted to discipline or terminate a client. Mr. Dana always said it wasn't about the clients doing something wrong. He always put it on the staff that they—the staff—were not doing their jobs correctly. He always said, "It isn't about the other person or situation, it is always about you and how you handle these things."

0

Mr. Dana went on: "Why is Tom Brady one of my role models? I'll tell you why. No one ever gave him a chance or thought he had a chance to make it as a professional football player. Never gave him a chance. He was a long shot, a huge underdog! Does that sound remotely familiar to any of you? No one *ever* believed in me, either, or gave me a fucking chance. Ever. I told all of you that I have sat in those same chairs you all sit in now, for God's sake. No one believed in me except *me*.

"One of the foundational tools I keep repeating is *believe*. Use it. Practice the class on words. That goes for all of you. You better *believe* in *yourself*; no one else does.

"Moving on, you had all these football executives, scouts, professionals making hundreds of thousands of dollars evaluating college players. They had simulators, computers, analysis graphs, and charts, and none of those so called 'professionals' thought Tom Brady had a chance. All those so called 'authorities' said Tom Brady was too slow,

152

couldn't throw a spiral, couldn't read the defense. One person finally took a chance and picked him . . . Tom was the one hundred and ninety-ninth pick. That means all those 'professionals' chose one hundred and ninety-eight people to play football before Tom Brady. That means all those 'professionals' thought those one hundred and ninety-eight other players were better than Tom Brady! None of those one hundred and ninety-eight are playing today. Tom Brady won a Super Bowl two years ago—his seventh! Playing for another team at the age of forty-three. Do you realize how difficult that is? Most football players *never, ever* play in a Super Bowl. Most players go their entire career without being in a Super Bowl. Tom Brady has played in ten!

0

Mac: Mr. Dana was speaking very forcefully and passionately while writing on the blackboard.

0

Mr. Dana went on: "With all the money that was spent to say Tom Brady wasn't good enough, there was one thing they missed, one problem: no machine, no computer, no expert could check Tom Brady's heart for *passion*! No 'expert' could put Tom Brady's desire on a machine and measure it. No one in or outside of football could talk Tom Brady into *not* believing in himself. My role model overcame difficult obstacles. My role model is a leader. My role model inspires others around him to be at their best and perform at their highest level. My role model refuses to ever settle. My role model never takes for granted his accomplishments or achievements.

"I'll tell you a quick story and then move on. After Tom Brady had won his fifth Super Bowl and the season was over, he called the core of his team a few weeks later. He said to his core teammates that he wanted all of them to meet at his ranch in Montana to practice. Now this is, like, two or three weeks after the season ended and the team won the Super Bowl. A few players said something like this: 'We just won the Super Bowl. I was going to take the family to the Caribbean or Hawaii.' Tom Brady said, 'That was last year. You want to win again? Practice, practice, practice. That's how you become a champion.' The team showed up in Montana to practice. By the way, they won another Super Bowl. True story."

0

Mac: Mr. Dana had written on the board "Champion, Practice, Desire, Passion, Motivator, Do Not Settle."

0

Mr. Dana pointed to the board and said, "Do you all see these words? I don't know Julian's grandfather, Sabrina's mom, or Anton's brother. I do not know Tom Brady. I *do* know how to be like them though. By applying these words into action every day of my life through disciplined practice.

"That's another foundational tool—discipline. I need all of you to notice how I use the words all the time that I have been teaching you daily by repeating them. Remember 'revolution'? Start overthrowing your old thoughts and talk. Start following role models. Those 'leaders' are what a role model is. A leader. You don't need to know them. All you have to do is follow their 'lead.' They have laid the path for you.

"Hey, Julian, do you ever complain?"

Julian shot back, "Fuck no! Never!"

Mr. Dana: "You see? Life is about following the leader. Not following the fucking loser!"

The class clapped until Mr. Dana motioned for them to stop.

Mr. Dana: "Another role model I do *not* know is Nelson Mandela. Mandela was a black activist born in South Africa. At the time, South Africa was under the rule of apartheid. Apartheid was a system of government in South Africa that favored racial segregation and favored whites. Blacks had a six to one majority in the population in South Africa, yet the whites ruled."

0

Mac: Mr. Dana had a way of telling a story with so much feeling that the class soaked it in. It was evident how much Mr. Dana believed in what he was saying. I think that is one of the main reasons clients flocked to him and respected him so much. The clients really believed in him.

0

Mr. Dana: "Mandela thought that was unfair and he protested. Mandela *rebelled*. There it is again, that word associated with revolution. Start putting these themes into all your thoughts and conversations. Anyway, Mandela was put in jail for twenty-seven years. Some of you, think about all of the time you've done. Mandela did twenty-seven years in a South African prison! The thing was, he never stopped dreaming of freeing South Africa. Mandela was beaten like a dog daily. Starved. Isolated. The white guards showed Mandela pictures of his wife making love to white men! My god, the torture he received daily. For twenty-seven years this went on. The horror.

"Nelson Mandela finally got out of prison. He freed South Africa from apartheid. He became the first black president of South Africa. Nelson Mandela won the Nobel Prize for Peace. They *could* *not* beat his *dream* out of him. They *could* *not* *stop* his desire and passion, even after twenty-seven years. Mandela freed a continent! Mandela freed a nation! Are you kidding me? After twenty-seven years of darkness, he freed a people! *They could not defeat his light!"*

0

Mac: Once again Mr. Dana was showing his intense passion. The class could see how much this man meant to Mr. Dana. They felt him!

0

Mr. Dana wrote more words on the blackboard and kept talking. "He freed a fucking *nation!*" Mr. Dana pointed to all the clients in a loud, confronting, challenging voice. "What do you all want? A fucking job? An apartment? A car? Your kids back? Boo-hoo-hoo. Mandela freed a *people* after being locked up for twenty-seven years. Remind me again why all of you are here. Remind me again what all of you keep saying you want. Free yourselves. Quit saying, 'It wasn't my fault.' Do something about it. Mandela freed a continent. This is how you do it."

Mr. Dana pointed to the blackboard and all the words describing a role model. "Be like Justin's grandfather. Stop complaining. Take responsibility for your actions and do something about it. Change it, for fuck sake."

Mr. Dana paused and then, in a soothing, calming

156

voice, he said, "Look, I get it. Everyone in here at one time or another in your young lives was dealt a shitty hand. You were forced to play those cards. But you are all here now due to the cards that *you* dealt *yourself* as an adult. Start dealing yourself winning cards. I have played a lot of poker. You *don't* need all aces to win. You *do* need to know how to read people and how to play your own cards the right way!

"I thank God for allowing me to speak to all of, and thank you for listening. Class is now over."

The class cheered and clapped before leaving the room.

Choice

"War Is just a shot away. Love is just a kiss away."

—The Rolling Stones

Mac: Mr. Dana came to class singing and dancing to the lyrics of "Gimme Shelter." The class was cheering as Mr. Dana did a few Jagger-like moves on the way to the podium. Mr. Dana shut off the music, took a bow to his clients' applause and started to speak in a cockney accent.

0

Mr. Dana: "Good evening and thank you for attending tonight's concert."

The class responded to this jovial mood with chants of, "More, more."

"Seriously, thank you all for joining me in class tonight. You all like music, of course. Let me see by a show of hands how many like Classical music. No one? Really? Country? Okay, about a third of the class. Hip Hop? Wow, almost all of you. Jazz? A few. Rock? Okay.

"So I see you have all decided which music appeals to you and which music you don't really care for. What you are actually doing is making a choice. Choice is simply making a decision when faced with two or more options or possibilities. Now look at the choices of music you all said you like just now. There is not a right or wrong choice. Some people don't like jazz. Some don't like heavy metal. Could someone tell me why they don't like Hip Hop? Leticia, go ahead."

Leticia: "I don't like all the ways it talks about women or what a lot of rappers say they do to women. I also don't like women rappers. I feel it degrades women like me who have fought for a bit of equality. It demeans women."

A few scattered boos rippled around the classroom.

Mr. Dana: " Knock your shit off or get the fuck out! Ms. Leticia has stated how she feels, and by jeering her you're saying her feelings don't matter. That's how that genre makes her feel. She *chooses* something different. It is her choice. It is her prerogative, her opinion.

"Now, some of you are smart enough to know where I'm going with this. She chooses something *different*.

"I cannot stand the taste of the energy drink Monster, but I love the green apple Rock Star energy drink. I choose something different. I am free to make this choice. Unfortunately, with addiction you are not free to choose something different. You all have to understand that when you are not free to make a choice, you become a slave. Of course, most of us, including me, can argue as an addict that, 'I *choose* to get high, to gamble, to watch porn all day, whatever.' Remember, as addicts, we are exactly like Picasso. But instead of being a painter, we are one of the greatest artists of justification and excuses. Most of us thought we were right.

"We did choose to watch porn all day or get high . . . at first. At first! Then what happened? After a while, you didn't have a *choice*, you lost your freedom to choose. Be honest, how many of you, before you chose to come in here, wanted to stop your addiction and could not? Raise your hands.

"Some of you are not being honest. If you could have stopped on your own, then why the fuck are you in here?

Please don't tell me the courts, CPS, your spouse, or some other bullshit like that made you come. It was already too fucking late. The bottom line is you *could not stop on your own*. You gave up your freedom of choice.

"Most of you . . . most were made to come here. I said a few of you were smart enough to choose before someone made you. That's the real truth. We have discussed countless times how your addiction made you a slave, stole your freedom. By stealing your freedom, your addiction robbed you of your free choice. The ability to choose. As addicts we gave that up.

"Now, by being here, you're earning your personal freedom back. You must focus on this and be aware of this. Fact: stay conscious of your decisions. Start asking yourself, 'Are my choices and actions in my best interests to move forward in life?'

"No one likes to be controlled. The human spirit likes to be in control of its own path. When you achieve true freedom from negative actions, negative decisions, and negative choices, your spirit will soar and know how to roam the earth. That is liberation. That is rediscovering what you and your life are really about. The liberation and freedom you obtain by making these *new choices* are an exercise for your soul. The positive, right choices are the equivalent of spiritual pushups. You might not be able to do many pushups today. Keep practicing. You are exerting energy in a positive way. The exercise is to continue those pushups until your body, mind, and spirit are in natural harmony . . . in balance. Isn't that what, deep down, you have been trying to fill with your addictions? The hollowness within. The issue is that instead of 'spiritual pushups,' you went the opposite way, you chose 'spiritual apathy.' Substitution and constitution— a new set of principles to live by. Your *choice*. That's the real truth, baby.

"I'm going to help you by showing you something about choices. Go back to the start of this lecture. I said, 'Choice is making a decision between two or more options.' Like music, energy drinks, etc., there are many choices to choose from.

"However, there are only three *life choices* you need to make to determine the direction of your life. There are no different options to choose from. There are *only* two absolute options in each of these three 'choices of life,' as I call them.

"Repeating myself again—and I do love hammering into your heads, oops, I mean reminding you of the past class on the purpose of obtaining new knowledge and being able to *think*. The more you hear and continue to absorb this new knowledge, the more you will start to think differently. When you think differently, you make new choices that change you for the better. Keep in mind, it is the ability to be more open minded that will allow you to expand your viewpoint. As addicts, we have a very narrow perspective on what information is allowed in our consciousness. Any information interfering with our addiction, regardless of whether the information is correct, is disregarded.

"When we were in our addictions and using the three life choices, the choice we constantly made the majority of the time was the wrong choice. Bear in mind that when you all leave here, the three life choices will no longer be influenced by your addictions. You will have regained your personal freedom. The freedom of choice. Determining which choice to make after the program should become instinctual, provided you truly, in your heart, desire recovery.

"The three life choices really just come down to Choice A or Choice B. There is nothing between A and B. This the only choice you can make with these choices of life:

A or B. Nothing else. Get your pencil or pen out and write this down."

Mr. Dana went to the blackboard and wrote:

The 3 CHOICES of LIFE

1: Any Choice you make will either:

A: HARM, HURT, or HINDER your Spiritual Growth

OR

B: HELP your Spiritual Growth

2: Any Choice you make will have:

A: CONSEQUENCES and PENALTIES

OR

B: REWARDS and BLESSINGS

3: Any Choice you make will lead to:

A: People CONTAMINATING and INFECTING YOU

OR

B: People ENRICHING and CONTRIBUTING to YOU

Mr. Dana walked back to the podium and continued: "These choices are so simple. As I have said and will always say, 'Simple does not mean easy.' When you continue to make these three choices of life, you reclaim your freedom. Think back to our first classes. Recovery means to regain what you lost. You lost your freedom and your power to choose the right choice. As I have preached from Day One that, 'The harder choice is always the right choice.' Making the right choice means you are not making the wrong choice. When you continually make the right choice, you are putting yourself on the road to your true destiny.

"By reclaiming your freedom, you are empowering yourself. Your spirit is becoming smarter, stronger, and more confident in controlling your own life and claiming your natural rights.

"I'm going to tell you a true story. I have a friend whose name is Cho-ee. I've known him for over forty years. Cho-ee is the greatest mechanic and biggest thief I have ever met. Anyway, when I first got clean, Cho-ee stayed an addict. Cho-ee would call me at, like, midnight or two a.m. and say, 'Man, come over right now and I can fix your brakes.' Now, I knew that if I went to Cho-ee's that late, I would most likely end up vacuuming the trunk at four in the morning and never getting to the brakes."

Mr. Dana had to wait as the class cracked up.

"Yeah, it's funny 'cause you all know what would have happened. As much as I love Cho-ee, I made the choice of not letting him contaminate or infect me.

"Cho-ee is clean going on five years now. However, he's still a thief. Getting clean does not take the asshole, thief, or liar out of you. You have to change your negative actions as well. Choice!

"Anyway, I still see Cho-ee, he works on my car and I've known him forty years. The other day I took him to Denny's, and when we got back in the car, he showed me all the silverware and salt and pepper shakers he stole. Fuckin' Cho-ee is still a thief."

The class laughed.

"On the way back from Denny's, I stopped at 7-Eleven for a Rock Star then I took Cho-ee home. When I got home I noticed all my quarters and my spare sunglasses had been taken from my glove box.

Fucking Cho-ee."

The class laughed.

"About two weeks ago my wife and I had to go to San Diego on a moment's notice. I asked Cho-ee if he could he turn on the lights, water my plants, and feed my dog while we were gone for a few days. Five days later, when we get home, my computer, TV, and plants were all gone. Cho-ee even stole my dog! Fucking Cho-ee! Whose fault is that? Mine or Cho-ee's?"

In unison, the class yelled, "Yours."

Mr. Dana, looking shocked: "Mine? Why?"

Most of the class yelled, "You knew Cho-ee was a thief."

One of the clients yelled, "Cho-ee couldn't help himself."

Another added, "You chose him to watch your house."

Mr. Dana: "Exactly. I *chose*. As you all said, Cho-ee could not help himself. I was free to choose. I did *not* follow and practice the three choices of life. I received *consequences*. A *penalty*. After the program, if one of your old friends is an alcoholic who always drinks, or a dope fiend who always has a pipe on them, always, always, always, and you decide to spend some time with the alcoholic or dope fiend, whose fault is it when you slip and relapse."

In one voice the class responded, "Mine."

Mr. Dana continued: "Your choice. Most likely you chose Option A in every one of the three life choices. I'm glad you all recognize it was your choice. No excuses. *Your choice*. Always practice the harder choice. Practice, practice, practice. As I said earlier, these three life choices become instinctual. Instinctual means automatic. Available without thinking. 'Just Do It,' as Nike says.

"Now when I came in to class, I wrote on the board

the line from the song 'Gimme Shelter' by The Rolling Stones. Regardless of whether or not you like the Stones, what does that line mean?"

Mr. Dana pointed to the blackboard. "Go ahead, Ms. Lydia."

Lydia: "Everyone has the choice of going to war or loving. Something like that."

Mr. Dana: "That's right. We have a simple choice of war or love. Remember when I told all of you that a hero was someone who saves lives?"

The class yelled, "Yes."

Mr. Dana: "A hero can also save situations and problems. Any of you ever have an argument with a spouse or family member? A boss? At the bank? What usually happens is that we are so busy losing focus on the bigger picture, we stay so narrow minded on the 'wanting to win' at that moment, that we end up going to war. 'War is only a shot away.' Think about arguing with your spouse. The smaller picture is something like, 'I don't like getting yelled at. My spouse is wrong and I am right.' So we choose to go to war. We argue, fight, get mad.

"Even if I win this war right now, which is this small, narrow moment, my spouse either slams the door, doesn't talk to me, or leaves. When I go to bed, my spouse sleeps in the other room or doesn't let me near her. This can go on for an hour, a day, it can even lead to relapse if you're the loser of this meaningless war. However, 'Love is only a kiss away.' It means be 'The Hero' of the situation. Instead of being a hero and saving lives, be the hero and save the situation! Use love in those situations. That is the choice: war or love. A or B. When I choose to become the hero of the situation, do you think my spouse sleeps on the couch? When I am the hero of the situation, do you think my spouse doesn't let me near her? Do you think any of us are mad, angry, slamming the door, or thinking about relapse? Fuck no!

"Save the situation by using love through making a *harder choice*. Words of love is a choice! This godly technique of choosing love works at the DMV, the bank, paying your bills, or when you're late paying a bill and you're facing a shut off. If you choose to go to war, do you think your service won't get turned off? I have told you all a thousand times that curtesy is the highest form of manipulation. And again, the harder choice is always the right choice. Is it *easy* to tell your spouse you're wrong? Fuck no. What's important to know and remember is that all conversation is a negotiation. Everyone has a motive . . . always. I have a motive with all of you. My motive is that I want you all to leave here new, better people. Motive is not a bad thing or a negative thing unless you're an addict or someone wanting something for yourself that isn't in your best interest. My motive is serving you.

"I want you to learn that not everyone knows how to communicate and say what they really mean, and the core truths get lost in the translation. I'm going to give you an example on becoming a proficient interpreter or translator.

"When I came out of rehab and went home, my wife said, 'If you ever use or drink again, I am going to throw all your shit out on the front lawn. I am going to change all the locks and then I am going to call the police.'

"Now, I was shocked. What I did, though, is I read between the lines. What I did was interpret and translate my wife's words. She really meant, 'I love you. If you get loaded again, I will die and it will kill the kids.' You see, at the time my wife *did not know* how to say those things. Lovers, family, friends, people in general do not always know how to say what they mean. Other people have their own limitations, their own issues, an inability to express real truth and real feelings. Understand, we are all simply people with our own personal struggles. Instead of always making each and everything always about you—that is addict thinking—start working on doing your best to understand the motive behind someone's inability to express themselves.

"Your job is to practice 'effective communication' and not go to war by making the wrong choice. Love is just a kiss away. Keep your focus always on your long-term personal goals. Most things are not going to matter in a month . . . why let them matter now? My wife and I have survived, struggled, loved each other for thirty-eight years. Now when we get heated at each other, one of us is the hero. We both laugh. Regardless of what an ass I can be most of the time."

The classed laughed.

"Yes, I said it. I can be an ass at times . . . or worse. I am no better than any one of you. I'm only farther along the path. I am teaching you the way to join me on this heavenly journey. Those who really practice, strive, put in the work, are going to pass me up and go farther than I could ever hope. Why? You have more time to learn and develop your spirit. I told all of you, I wasted thirty-five years of my life going the bent, crooked way.

"Anyway, getting back to my wife and my laughing now in tight moments. We laugh, as we both know that when we go to bed at night we want to hold each other. We know that, in the morning, we each want to wake up smiling to ourselves and each other. Most importantly, we know that in a week it isn't going to matter. If it really is not a life-changing incident affecting our lives, it's not worth expending energy and, more importantly, our valuable time on meaningless bullshit. Learn to analyze situations. Stop reacting; that's addictive thinking and behavior. Foreign language and customs. Remember that class? Use your classes together and create 'instinctual synergy.' Instill within yourself the conviction that 'if it won't really matter later, don't let it matter now.'

"This new knowledge needs to be instilled in your instinctual core to avoid any personal wars. You have to approach each day with a sense of determination to pay attention and grow your spirit. When you go to bed, you *must* be better than when you woke up. That means when you wake up each morning, you are ready to do all and everything you can to be better. Not better than anyone else, just better than *you* were the day *before*.

"It is imperative that you always pay attention to your thoughts. Your thoughts transform into action. Your actions morph into habits. Habits create character. *Your* character. Character means what kind of person are you. If your thoughts are about seeking your addiction, that will form into negative actions. When your negative actions consistently bring you into your addiction, it becomes a negative habit. Then your character is one of negativity. Negative character can be lying, cheating, sneaking, stealing, hateful, angry, violent, whatever. You all know what type of negative character you had in your addictions.

"Oh yeah, I forgot to mention that after you have achieved negative character, that negative character forms, cements, guarantees one thing. Anyone know what that is? Go ahead, Leonard."

Leonard: "Uh, death?"

Mr. Dana: "Yep. Anyone else? Sofie?"

Sofie: "Homelessness or prison?"

Mr. Dana: "That's right. We have homelessness, prison, death. In other words, your negative character morphs into your negative *destiny*. In other words, *character* transforms into *destiny*, which is another word for your future. You are here to change your future! You're all here, aren't you? Negative destiny. Mr. Ian, can I ask you how old you are?"

Ian: "Mr. Dana, you know I'm nineteen."

Mr. Dana: "You married?"

Ian: "C'mon, Mr. Dana, you know I'm not."

Mr. Dana: "Yes, Ian, I know all that, but I wanted everyone in here to know it. Ian is nineteen. It's a hundred and five degrees out in this desert. It's summertime. Your *negative destiny* is here right now. My God . . . Ian, you're nineteen. You're almost good looking. I said *almost*. I don't want to say Ian's good looking; it will only go to his head."

The class all laughed.

Mr. Dana: "You should be up at the lake on jet skis. You should be at the beach, watching chicks playing volleyball in their bikinis. Drinking root beer floats. What the fuck, man. You should be living the dream of youth. Not smoking fucking meth.

"Ian, you hurt my soul. My soul aches for you and everyone in here who isn't doing all they can to change the direction of their lives. All you older men who fucked up your youth should be telling Ian the real truth.

"This recovery program is the only thing I can think of that starts out as a negative consequence based on your negative actions and habits and can transform you into receiving a positive blessing. Of course, this is only based on if you are practicing positive thoughts and actions in the program today! Choice. Your *choice*.

"The beauty and good news for Ian *and* the rest of you is that this principal works in reverse. Positive thoughts to positive action, positive action to positive habits, positive habits transform into positive character. And then a fucking *positive destiny*! *Give* to *get*. Class is now adjourned."

The entire class whooped and laughed as they filed out.

Q & A and Additional Thoughts

Mac: Mr. Dana told me earlier that he was going to open the class up to questions from the clients. Mr. Dana said he was always asked so many questions between classes and after classes that he was going to run today's session based on clients' questions and Mr. Dana's own thoughts on a range of subjects. I was looking forward to this, as I enjoyed and learned from these interactions. Mr. Dana was way early and already at the podium, reading a book, as the class came in to take their seats.

0

Mr. Dana: "Hello, class. Today, we're going to do something different. Today is going to be Mr. Dana's Asked and Answered. Meaning you can ask me almost any question as long as it's done with absolute respect. You can object to my opinion and voice your own. If you don't like my opinion, don't worry about it. I'll get even with you later."

The class laughed.

"No, really, ask away. The questions I will not answer or answer in a diffused or abstract way are personal ones that focus on my family. I hope you all can understand and respect that. Being a teacher and counselor, the focus should not be about me anyway. The teaching and focus should always be for and on you clients. Please, remember, be respectful, I don't want to jump all over you. The way we do this is that you raise your hand and I'll call your name and you can shoot me a question. Let's do this thing."

0

Mac: The class seemed a little bit intimidated to ask questions. I had learned after all these weeks getting to know the clients that it was due to their respect for Mr. Dana and not wanting to sound stupid in front of him. What's interesting is that Mr. Dana always, always tells the clients they are so much smarter than almost anyone in the facility or in his life. And he meant it.

0

Ian was the first to be acknowledged by Mr. Dana. Ian asked, "When did you really know you were an addict? I mean, how did you know you were really addicted?"

Mr. Dana: "I knew when I would go to the casino with a hundred dollars to play the dollar slots. I would put the hundred in the machine and play one hand for a hundred dollars instead of the one-dollar-a-hand game a hundred times. I knew I was an addict when I bought a bottle of liquor so I could have *one* drink. I would have that one drink . . . and then drink the *entire* bottle. I really knew I was an addict when the directions on my Percodan prescription said to take one pill every hour hours, and I would take eight pills every hour. I didn't need anyone to tell me I was an addict. You see, I self-diagnosed. My diagnosis was called 'Addictive Dyslexia.'

The class burst out laughing.

Miss Georgina was next. She asked, "Can you give us examples when, during your addiction, you were the most scared you have ever been? And what scares you now?"

Mr. Dana: "Sure, I've reflected on that a number of times. During my addiction, when my youngest daughter had major surgery, I trembled, trembled horribly with fear. I was so scared; I had no faith in anything. If you recall I said that addicts are movie stars. We are always acting. In the

172

hospital, my script was taken away and I wasn't in control of anything . . . except the bill, which I most likely never paid. Also, countless times my fear roared up when was working in the film industry and I couldn't support my family. I was broke. I mean as broke as anyone could possibly be, with no one to tell my fears to, no one I could tell how scared I really was. I couldn't ask anyone—family or even friends—for money. I didn't have any of those foundational tools we've talked about. I never, deep down, *believed* in myself, had any *faith* in myself, or faith in a Higher Power. And what scares me now? My wife!"

The class laughed again.

"Seriously, today, I really don't have any fears. That is the fucking truth. If I have some huge problem or big issue, I don't run to it. I let it come to me. By the time it gets to me, it's not so big anymore. God has got me."

Ms. Georgina: "Could you explain letting problems come to you?"

Mr. Dana: "Let me give you a visual analogy. All of you, picture this. You're at the beach and the waves are huge. I mean ten feet, twenty feet. If I swim out to those huge waves, they're going to flip me, knock me under, take my breath away, or even drown me. However, when I stand on the edge of the water and I see that huge wave, I let it come to me. By the time it gets to me, I've had time to decide if I want to jump over it, go through the wave, ride it in, or back up. Usually, a twenty-foot wave is about one foot by the time it gets to my feet. It's the same wave. The same exact wave. But now it's way smaller and a hell of a lot less powerful. Call it 'perspective analyzation.'"

Lewis: "What is your religion? You've quoted from the Bible, the Koran, Buddhist teachings . . . but you've never told us your religion."

Mr. Dana: "I don't have a religion. Keep in mind, this

is my opinion. Every religion I have ever studied has some of the same elements or threads running through them to help anyone be a better spiritual being on earth. I look at each religion as separate branches on a tree trunk. Some tree branches are sturdier, some thicker, some thinner than others. Every single branch, thin or thick, at the top or the bottom, all come from the tree trunk. For me, that tree trunk from which all the different branches grow is the 'Creator of all the Creation.' That is what I base my spirituality on. The tree trunk."

Ronaldo: "I relapsed, as you know. I know I stopped practicing all my tools. However, even practicing the tools, I got bored."

Assorted class voices called out, "Me, too." "Boredom." "Yeah, being bored."

Ronaldo continued: "How do you overcome boredom?"

Mr. Dana: "I'm not insulting any of you. Keep that in mind. As I have said, these are only *my* opinions. One thing to remember about my opinion is that my opinions get me home at peace every night. Your opinions got you in this fucking place." Mr. Dana gestured at the facility, looked around at the ceiling and out the windows.

0

Mac: Wow! Mr. Dana wasn't pulling any punches. He was leaning against the podium, so very relaxed. Usually, he was pacing and animated. But today, he was so matter of fact . . . like chatting to a friend.

0

Mr. Dana: "When I hear someone saying they're bored, what

they're actually saying—and I'm using the tool 'all conversation is a negotiation' from the Choices class—is that they're boring to themself. There are five hundred TV channels, the internet, X boxes, VR, Tic Tock, drones, radio cars. Fuck, man, I only had two channels on a black-and-white TV when I was growing up. But I had this"—he pointed to his head—"an imagination. Sticks and dirt. Every one of you have so much. If you're bored, go be of service. Yeah, I know, boring . . . and you can be right at times. Practice and use the tools of your 'library.' Ronald, you picked the two books the librarian said you could not read. Those two books always end the same. You've read them. The real truth is that you cannot be alone with yourself and your personal thoughts. You're always wondering, 'What is he or she doing? I need to go over here or there.'

"This boredom, as you all call it, is you running and escaping from yourself. You got into your addictions with others so you didn't have to be alone. You did not like what you were thinking about. I want to repeat this: in your addiction you did not like the voice in your head, your self-talk. You could not stand being by *yourself.* Then you got so far into your addiction that you didn't care anymore about yourself, so you isolated. Your true voice was so quiet, almost dead.

"You all need to learn to be your own best friend. All of you in here are practicing self-care. You're learning in here to care for your physical, mental, and spiritual self. When you leave here, continue to do these classes, especially the daisy/spirit class as I have taught you. Self-care turns into self-love. When I'm home alone, I'm with my best friend."

Mr. Dana started kissing his hands and everyone in the room laughed. "I dig where my mind is at. How can I ever be alone again? I have my best friend with me all the time now and"—he pointed upward—I have God. Bored?

Are you fucking kidding me? I'm at peace. Sometimes, I just sit and dig my imagination, dig my thoughts, good or bad. All of you over time will learn to enjoy being with yourself. Then you won't be bored. Learn to love yourself. Then you won't run away from yourself; you will always want to be with your best friend—*you*."

Ms. Ariana: "You have said to go to ninety meetings in ninety days. But you just said meetings can be boring. Isn't that a contradiction?"

Mr. Dana: "You are one hundred percent correct. Go to ninety meetings in ninety days. And yes, meetings are sometimes worse than boring. Look, when I got out of the program, I would wake up at five a.m., take a shower, go to the AM/PM get my coffee and my Monster drink, exactly like everyone else did and still does. I would get to my little meeting room behind my church and go in at six a.m. sharp. At times, I would be with only one other person. Sometimes, there were two, three, or four people, and it would still be a boring meeting. Other times, it could be a good, really insightful meeting with five people in attendance. Or maybe it was only me and the one guy who unlocked the door at five fifty-nine a.m. But I went go to that meeting every day. And you know what? Some days, the guy who had the commitment to unlock the door would not show up at all. I would sit in the parking lot, smoking, waiting for the guy, for a half hour and then then leave.

"I learned it wasn't about the meeting. It was about me committing to myself, it was about that foundational tool of 'Relentless Commitment' and going to a meeting. If the guy didn't show up, I still felt great—the foundational tool of 'Self-Motivation.' I had the power to make myself feel great. If the guy showed up and the meeting was boring, I still felt great. If the meeting was insightful, not only did I feel great, I had some new insight into myself or my

176

recovery. The meetings are always about proving yourself to you. Remember the class on 'the chip on the shoulder.' I proved to myself in those early days that I was serious about changing my life. I went to *three meetings a day for ninety fucking days*! That's the real truth.

"It wasn't because I was bored or thought I would go get loaded. It was that I had wasted so much time in my addiction, as you all know. Again, I was proving something to *me*. I was learning to show myself how much I cared for myself by wanting to change. That's how you fall in love with yourself again. Doing wonderful things to your spirit. Each meeting, each commitment, each harder choice are those 'exercises for the soul.' I put my *all* into my recovery. You all see the fucking result," he said and pointed to himself. "Thank you, God!"

The class erupted in cheers.

Ms. Carissa: "Mr. Dana, you're always repeating we should speak from the heart to someone else's heart. Go A to B. The 'real truth.' Do you always tell the real truth?"

Mr. Dana: "Fuck, no. I lie."

The class laughed.

Mr. Dana: "Look, I'm conscious of lying. I'm not perfect. I'm always, constantly, in a state of spiritual repair or spiritual renovation. The truth to the trained ear sounds so beautiful . . . like the sound of Himalayan windchimes made of crystal. To those who are on the way to learning to 'walk with giants,' you hear those truthful 'windchimes.' Even without any wind! To those who live in *truth*, they hear the loud clanking of a cowbell every time someone lies to them. Clank, clank, *clank*. That's what a lie sounds like. Truth has such a beautiful sound. Nothing can stand up to God's tools. Truth. Love. Honesty.

"You see, when we lie, deceive, hate, whatever, all those 'dark tools' actually do protect the spirit.

177

Unfortunately, they are protecting in an ungodly way. The problem is that those 'dark tools' are like leaden armor. You know, that shit like the bomb squad wears? It's hard to move around in that leaden armor. It's bulky, clumsy, thick. It does protect you though. Using 'dark tools' keeps all things from entering our soul from the outside. It is an impenetrable protection. So you're protecting your spirit, as nothing can get in and touch it. The bigger problem is that by having this protection, as I said, *nothing gets in.* Nothing goes out either. Your spirit just sits in a blinded, self-imposed exile. Your true spirit is locked, stunted, waiting, shrinking, starving behind those impenetrable bars of isolation.

"God's tools are like the Himalayan wind. Bright, fresh, free, crystal clear. You feel it, you know it's there, and it's invisible. It is *not* heavy, leaded, bomb-squad material. Put another way, God's tools are like a *Star Wars* force field: invisible. A to B from the heart. Pure protection. On this invisible wind, nothing gets in except for truth and love. Nothing goes out except truth and love. That's spirituality in its highest form."

Ms. Carissa: "It hurts to hear some things that are true when said by others. It also hurts at times even if things aren't true. Lies hurt as well."

Mr. Dana: "I'm going to answer that in the reverse. Everyone here as always been told that the 'Truth hurts.' Why is that?" Mr. Dana walked across the class and back to the podium. "I guess from way over here, I'm going to hurt you and steal your joy by saying a mouthful of lies, call you all sorts of horrible, horrible names. You said that lies hurt you at times. The reason is that you haven't learned how to protect your spirit. Most of us can protect ourselves from a physical punch. Most of us can keep someone from stealing our wallet or purse. Learn to use God's tools. Learn how to block lies from hitting your soul. Learn how to keep words

178

from stealing your joyful spirit. That is you in charge of controlling yourself. Empowerment. Not to let others control us or have power over us.

"The way we learn is to listen for the truth from others. Learn to tell the truth, be honest, learn to *choose,* use the tool 'a kiss away.' When you learn to do these things, then no one can hurt you or steal your joy from across the room again. You will have a *Star Wars* force field around you. It is never, ever about the other person, regardless of how nasty, evil, or cruel they can be. It is always, in any circumstance, about you. *Do your job.* Keep practicing these tools of God that are imbedded in your breath and being. Nothing stands up to God's tools. I mean, they're God's. They're *pure.*

"Addiction cannot stand up to God. I told all of you awhile back that addiction does not care if you're young or old. Rich or poor. Black or white. Men, women, or both."

Mr. Dana waited for the laughter to die down and then continued: "Addiction is one of the least prejudiced things you will ever encounter. Addiction cares about one thing only—killing your spirit. The only thing God wants is for your spirit to shine, not hide in the dark shadows, running from yourself. God's tools always win out.

"Now before taking another question, let me finish up with 'the truth hurts.' Instead of always thinking about yourselves like addicts, understand that the person who tells someone the truth gets hurt as well. It hurts *me* to tell *you*— or someone I really care about—the truth. It hurts the truth teller. That is why the truth hurts."

Frankie: "Sir, as you know, I'm going to leave here soon. I haven't had a job since I was seventeen. I'm twenty-six now. All I ever did to make money was hustle and sell dope. How do I tell the truth on my resume? Or what about the job skills part? Should I list my skills as able to steal, sell dope, and run fast?"

The class cracked up.

Mr. Dana: "You worked in the kitchen here, didn't you? You were on the volleyball team. You did extra chores when some of you here thought you were fooling the staff by not doing your assignments. I'm glad some of you realized that was your addiction making you fool and cheat yourselves. Once you understood that, you have stepped up your chores.

"Frankie, you've been starting to feel proud by showing yourself discipline, showing yourself hard work. Frankie, feeling proud for a job well done, discipline, and hard work are great job skills. In the kitchen you were able to follow orders, do more than one job, serve crappy food—and it is crappy—without arguing with the staff, the head of the kitchen, or the clients when they bitched and moaned about the food. Those are wonderful attributes called 'soft job skills.' On your resume, maybe think about putting 'able to follow orders,' 'multi-tasking,' and 'positive communication.' In volleyball you learned to be a team player, able to stand, do physical exercise without complaint. You kept score, didn't you? That's 'math skills.' You cheered your team on and believed in winning as a team. That would be 'teamwork' and 'goal oriented.' Something along those lines. Doing extra chores shows a 'willingness to take on extra challenges' and 'doing more than assigned work.' I mean that is the truth. You did those things.

"Frankie, every day, all day, you come up to me and ask me a litany of questions. Every day. The number one thing employers are looking for today isn't a college diploma. That's what used to be the 'gold standard.' Today, employers want to see how curious you are, how interested you are in obtaining more knowledge. That is a fact. Start looking at the positive things you're doing for yourself. Your addictive thinking makes you look at negativity in yourself and is always reminding you of your failures.

"I'm going to show all of you something." Mr. Dana went to the blackboard and started writing with his back to the class while speaking.

0

Mac: As I was always seated facing the class, I usually stared at Mr. Dana's back. He was now facing me. His back was to the class while he wrote. He gave me a wink and a smile. He was up to something.

0

Mr. Dana: "Look, recovery is a simple math problem." You see, truth"—as Mr. Dana wrote on the blackboard, he spoke the words:

TRUTH. 2 x 1 = 2. Simple math.
HONESTY. 2 x 2 = 4. Simple math.
LOVE. 2 x 3 = 7.
You see? Simple math.
FAITH 2 x 4 = 8. Simple.
SELF. 2 x 5 = 10.

Mr. Dana turned back to the class. "So simple."

The class was laughing and whispering, and Mr. Dana asked,

"What? What's up? Why are you all fidgety and whispering? Someone, tell me what's up, please. Is my fly open? What's going on?"

Ryan: "Mr. Dana, you multiplied wrong."

Mr. Dana did not turn back to the blackboard. He said, "Look, I know how to do simple multiplication. I don't make mistakes. You all know that."

Various clients in class yelled, "Yes, you did." "You made a mistake." "Two times three is six. You put seven."

Mr. Dana turned, looked at the blackboard, and circled his mistake. "Fuck, you're all correct. I did make a mistake. However, why didn't any of you say, 'Mr. Dana, you got four out of five right.' All of focused on my mistake, my failure.

"Let me tell all of you something. I will take four out of five winning blackjack hands. I will take four out of five winning numbers in the lotto. I will take four out of five correct answers on the DMV test. I'll take four out of five dollars. Why didn't anyone here say, 'Mr. Dana, you got four out of five right.' Why did all of look at my error?

"That is your addictive thinking pattern. Shit, if I want to find mistakes, I could tell you all day what's wrong with each staff member, what's wrong with this facility, what's really wrong with the cafeteria food, what's wrong with all of you. In a heartbeat. Shit. I look for what is *right* in everything. Stop looking at the one out of five, the mistake . . . the failure. That's addictive, negative thinking. You need to be aware of that all the time. Concentrate on the four out of five that are right. Imagine looking at yourselves all day, every day, always looking at the one out of five in you! No wonder you can't be alone with yourself. No wonder you're bored. No wonder your self-esteem is shot. You all look at the one out of five inside yourselves. Instead, look at the four out of five inside each of you. Look at your successes. Your beauty always, always, always outshines your failures and ugliness. Unless your failures and ugliness are so big that they outshine your beauty. No one looks at the flaw in a diamond ring. Whenever anyone shows us a diamond ring, we always say, 'How much?' or 'It's beautiful.' We look at the brilliance, the facets, not the flaws."

Mr. Dana had to wait as the class clapped relentlessly. Then, laughing, he continued: "And by the way, you really don't think I know what two times three really is?"

The class laughed and applauded.

0

Mac: I was stunned and amazed.

0

Mr. Dana: "Next question please."

Ms. Carla: "Mr. Dana you always stress positive communication. You don't allow swearing in class or anywhere on campus. Why then do you get to swear? I mean, is that because you're Mr. Dana? You're looked up to here, and to a lot of us you're our role model."

The class cried out, "Yeah. Why?"

Mr. Dana: "Oh, you are so right. I'm not going to make any excuses. I do swear a little bit in class. However, all of you swear all the time. I hear you on the phone, in the smoke pit, with each other, and it's due to the fact that most of you don't have any other vocabulary. The truth hurts, remember that."

Mr. Dana changed his easy bantering style and now employed a professional, fast-talking voice. "When I talk to your parole agents, CPS workers, families, do you think I swear? When I go to the county meetings to improve this program or seek a grant, do you think I swear? I happen to have an extensive vocabulary, I'm able to enunciate when I'm expressing my point of view. I can elaborate on a myriad

183

of subjects with a depth and knowledge in which most people would be lost or need a dictionary to understand and communicate with me on an intellectual level. In addition I also possess the ability to listen closely and respond when needed to the appropriate subject being discussed. Furthermore . . ."

The class erupted in clapping.

Mr. Dana's voice returned to friendly bantering. "Furthermore, I feel that swearing at times can emphasize the effect, tone, and subject matter in these classes. The swear words I use, after all, are in the English language. Ms. Carla is right though. Thank you, Carla. I'm going to try . . . no, I'm gonna actually *do*. You all see, that's another class we all attended. Always incorporate your tools daily. Ms. Carla, I will cut down on my swearing in class. Thank you for the constructive criticism. Of course, see me after class, as you have extra chores and assignments."

The class again cracked up.

Ms. Carla: "One last, follow-up question, please. How do you read between the lines when it comes to what you said about 'all conversation is a negotiation?'"

Mr. Dana: "All you have to do is identify what that person is saying. Then understand the person and why they're saying it. When I can do that, I am able to manage *my* response and not just react. I have always preached that it is never about the other person, the problem, the issue, whatever. It is *always* about *you* and responding to those things. I do my best to stay balanced on 'higher ground.' I do my best to *not* get sucked down into others' lack of knowledge or bullshit. It's easier to let go. Not waste any more of my time. That not easy at all, though. It takes practice. The real truth is that's the main area I'm personally working on. Identify. Understand. Manage. That's the ground floor of emotional intelligence. That cannot be done until you accept who you are and truly get real with yourself. You working on your 'controlling of self' in a positive way, including your thoughts.

"I don't imagine anyone can be a 'translator' for other people's conversations until they can clearly identify and understand their own thoughts, emotions, and actions, both good and bad, and then manage them. Only then can you be what I call an 'interpreter' or 'translator' of others.

"I can take two more questions, as we are way over on time."

Rinaldo: "Mr. Dana, I ain't embarrassed about it. Most people in here know anyways. You taught me to read two months ago. Remember? You made me read Dr. Seuss out loud to you every day. *The Sneetches* was the name of the book. You said that in order to get comfortable with talking, I needed to read out loud every day. You said it would also make me a better reader. I want to know what I need to do to get more intelligent and smarter."

Mr. Dana: "Great question. Thank you for asking that. First, I recommend to all of you in here to read aloud a minimum of fifteen minutes every day. I don't care if it's from the 'Good Book,' the 'Big Book,' a cookbook, or a comic book. Get comfortable hearing yourself. Reading aloud makes you self-confident when speaking to others. It builds self-assurance, which includes self-esteem. Self-esteem is how I feel about myself. When I have confidence, when I feel good about myself, I gain self-value. In other words, I am worth more to myself. That is self-worth. You've all seen people with a 'vibe.' 'Vibe' comes from 'vibrations.' Some people have this vibrance, a force of energy, a self-assuredness. They walk into a room and we are immediately attracted to them.

"Look at it from a scientific point of view. Atoms collide, creating energy and fusion. Fusion *within* powers our Sun. When atoms keep bouncing into each other, it creates so much atomic power that it becomes radioactive, like our Sun. Nuclear bombs are made from splitting atoms and bouncing them back at each other, and when these atoms collide, they 'trigger' a powerful explosion. The God particle is a perfect example. Scientists at the Cern Laboratory in Switzerland are using lasers to shoot particles at each other at the highest speeds along an underground, twenty-six-mile track. When those atoms hit each other, creation of pure energy turns to creating the brightest light. That is science.

"Now, I'll use 'spiritually' in place of 'science' under the same conditions. Look at the 'self.' If you can use all the 'self' to bounce at each other like atoms, you will create the God particle within yourself and shine bright like the Sun. When you have self-confidence, it 'triggers' self-esteem, as I said earlier. Self-worth collides like an atom into self-value. This creates energy and now I have self-respect. When I have self-respect, my self-value goes up. Now I have *myself*, which includes self-trust, self-care, self-love, self-assessment, self-inspiration, self-improvement, self-discovery, self-respect, on and on, like a chain of atoms. That's simply science applied on the spiritual plane.

"It is for that scientific reason—or I should say spiritual principle—that I have been urging all of you to use all of those foundational tools combined—and they *must* be used together. Foundational tools used together create a spark. Add that first spark to your affirmations and they combine into a bigger spark. The ignition of your energy has been started. Science shows that a star's energy does not go out. When a star is going out, it burns the brightest. Your energy will continue to glow, your soul will shine and burn forever. It is called 'spiritual illumination.'

That energy—or spiritual illumination—attracts

positivity into our lives. Exactly like the Sun's gravity. I apologize to Paula Abdul and her song "Opposites Attract." No, they fucking don't! Positivity attracts positivity. Love attracts love. We are magnets; we attract things into our orbit. Exactly like the Sun.

"Remember, though, there is both a negative and positive charge in atoms. It works in reverse as well. When I don't have self-confidence, it collides into self-misery and creates an ongoing, negative chain reaction. Instead of 'shining bright,' you are dark, etcetera. Exactly like the death of a star. A star that dies creates a black hole. It sucks everything into darkness. When we collide negative atoms within ourselves, we suck everything dark and negative into our beings. We turn self-ugly, self-hated, self-angered, self-disrespected. The opposite of love. We are magnets and we attract in this state of *death*, not *life*. Addicts die. There's another class. I don't want to dwell on this. You all can figure out how 'dark self' is the addictive particle. Me, I prefer the brightness within of the God particle. "

0

Mac: Mr. Dana was really rolling. I knew this was his favorite subject. I also knew he would make his point and cut this short. I still remember paying for a ticket right after the program to see him do a seminar on this theme called "Perfection and Energy of the Universe In Our Daily Lives." He loved using the Sun and planets orbiting around it perfectly to make an example of our lives. I have it in my original notebook from six years ago. There are two to four billion stars in our Milky Way galaxy. Each of these billions of stars have orbiting planets doing exactly the same thing as our planets do. They go around their suns in a precise, rhythmic pattern. Then to add to this that there are two to four billion galaxies, each with two to four billion stars. The planets going around the stars, the stars going around in their own separate galaxies, the galaxies going around each other in the Universe. New star clusters being born, dark stars with black holes dying, all doing this "cosmic ballet" to precision.

Mr. Dana was doing the same thing. Creating energy from within himself, using the clients as the planets attracted to his gravity. He was weaving a magic carpet for all to ride out of their addictions. I wonder, is this the "One-way ticket out of the hell of addiction" that he always talked about?

0

Mr. Dana: "Rinaldo, you have reading aloud as the first thing to do. The second thing I would do is to study the Universe. You don't need to read Stephen Hawking. Look at photos of the Sun, galaxies, supernovas, the planets, other phenomenon. Go online and type in 'Hubble Space photos,' 'Nasa photos,' or 'sun and star photos.' When you understand the basic principles of the 'Creation of the Universe' from the 'Maker of the Tree Trunk' that I talked earlier about, you will see how perfect God truly is. Remember, God is always giving hints and clues; lift your head to the heavens for the biggest hint and clue.

"Last question."

Ms. Jaz: "Why did you become a counselor?"

Mr. Dana: "Well, I guess, as I told Frankie earlier, it was because of curiosity. I was curious, after I got clean, to figure out the 'how' in my addiction. I studied, breathed, examined myself, and addictions in general. I looked at every angle of myself. I studied addiction from up close, far away, over, beneath, in between, whatever. I found my answer regarding my addiction. The answer was quite simple. I was a fucking, stubborn idiot. I never listened to those 'in the know.' My addictive voice of personal failure within was too strong.

"However, now 'I know' and so do all of you. Learn and listen, don't be like I was . . . unwilling to listen. Also, I get paid . . . not a lot though, but I get to talk to all of you, for which I receive the 'Divine Dividend' from above. God's plan is perfect. All the shit I've been through to end up here. The bad times, good times. God put me here in front of all of you. Right here, right now. Think about it. I'm dancing to the cosmic ballet.

"I am so honored to talk with all of you. Thank you. Class is fucking over. Oops, sorry, Ms. Carla, I'll work harder on my language."

The class whooped in unison and then filed out of the room.

SPIRITUALITY

GetOffDrugs

There is only "The one true way" to rid anyone of their addictive nature, negativity, and morally erroneous choices that lead to personal disaster. The one true way is based around the spiritual connection between the individual and the "Creator of the Creation." For the purpose of understanding for myself and all others, I will refer to this spiritual connection as God. As mentioned earlier, this spiritual connection within any individual can only be described as the *real truth*. The real truth of having the instinctual consciousness and reflexes of knowing right from wrong and good over bad. This "instinctual consciousness" is present within all human beings when born and is consistently being evolved and developed when nurtured along with daily, constant teachings.

I have often wondered when and where I, along with others, began to veer as well as wander way off the path of instinctual purpose and growth of the spirit. I have realized I was not born or placed on this planet for the progression of negative thoughts and actions to create misery and darkness in my life. I was not put on earth to despise myself and use tools of deception to accomplish what I thought were lofty goals.

These traits were *learned* negative behaviors. I had to learn and be tutored by example from fraudulent mentors in my life, along with teaching myself how to hate, lie, cheat, deceive, steal, deny, etcetera. Through daily and on-going practice, I progressed from proficiently familiar to deep intimacy with all learned negative behaviors, including negative thinking patterns and actions. The combined result of these negative tutorials and lessons led to my embracing the dark side of life. Welcoming this lifestyle of dark living allowed me to abandon all my God-given instinctual moral traits, along with disregarding any concept of personal integrity. With the acquisition and daily usage of these ungodly traits and habits, I distanced my conscious, spiritual being from myself. By ignoring it, in combination with the lack of exercise of this divine, spiritual connection, the result was stagnation and failure of growth of the spiritual human being. What was created and manifested "within self" was a dark, deep void, lacking in and of any spiritual existence.

The human being is not meant to walk the earth untethered from God. By walking untethered from God's compass, the spiritual being's instinctual consciousness falls out of calibration. Without godly calibration, the spirit within is lost. Struggling mightily, while searching to escape this dark void, the spirit condemns itself because of the lack of God's calibration. The spirit's desire to feed on evolutionary growth is an ongoing, diminishing prospect. The spirit's inability to feed itself through love of self, love of all others, lack of hard, moral decisions, and personal integrity leaves the spirit starving. Love, purpose, and meaning create purified education, along with balance on earth, for one's own spirit. Lacking harmonic balance, the only option left for the spirit to feed on and fill up this dark void is the pursuit and the obtaining of negative achievements. This includes the greatest achievement of all . . . the mastery and enslavement of the spirit through addiction.

This is the darkest, most evil existence one can create for one's "self." This is one of the main reasons why every addict is rushing to extinguish their light. It is the reason every addict sells their souls, mortgages their futures, eventually finding temporary residency in addiction. The addict is fully aware they are not fulfilling their spiritual contract with God. Through negative behaviors, thoughts, and actions, the human being is moving away from God. The human being is not walking in *truth*.

The addict has altered the course of the spirit's real purpose and is following an uncalibrated compass to their death. The addict finds identity, purpose, and meaning through negative thoughts, negative actions, and negative behaviors. This false identification allows the addict to become something they truly were not destined to be. The addict becomes morally out of tune and, through the corruption of personal self-value, is willing (albeit, rather reluctantly) to sell their soul for the addiction and accompanying behaviors. The end result of this bargain or contract is spiritual erosion, emotional homicide, and an amputation of one's dreams and desires to live in harmonic balance.

The addict finds a flitting, temporary reprieve of "filling what is missing" through the addiction process. However, this temporary reprieve is not the fulfilling, lifetime answer of what is missing in their life. The addict is painfully and acutely aware that what is missing is God's love.

The addict is reluctant to admit to others and to themselves that they have ventured down the wrong path. They know, in the deepest parts of their spiritual being, that they are wrong. Dead wrong. The addict embraces a walk so far away from the real truth of God's love. The real truth *is* God's love. That is the only answer to the addict's ongoing hunt for finding "what is missing." The addict continues this long, spiraling, downward, dead-end search with countless stops to fill this deepest of voids within self through the addiction process. Unbeknownst to the addict, God's love stimulates love of self, purpose, and meaning with a foundation based on the principles of purity.

This godly foundation is initially constructed using the materials provided by God, which consist of faith and hope. Eventually, the strongest of all foundations is built upon with the evolution of spiritual tools. These "tools" are in constant transformation based on personal usage. As the spirit masters the tools of God, which largely consist of love, kindness, truth, hope, honesty, gratitude, giving, and peace, the internal construction and upward growth of the soul increases toward God and is heaven bound.

Unfortunately, the close-minded addict is busy developing and building a foundational structure based on the premise of fear and hopelessness while being fully aware of its eventual collapse and demise. Regardless, this does not hinder or stop the addict, who continues to build on this condemned foundation. In addition the addict is totally aware of the eventual collapse of what is being built. This is contrary to the spirit's quest of obtaining healthy growth based on the "instinctual consciousness" God provides in each individual.

In time the addict's foundation, and all the addict has built on top of this flawed foundation, crumbles, leaving the addict with a dilemma. The addict has only two options to consider. Option #1 consists of a minor or major rebuild based on the amount of damage to the addict's poorly designed foundation. This decision is formed from the composition compiled of denial, untruths, and excuses. By employing these negatives and listening to the loud, non-stop, persistent calling of the addiction, along with a blinding, closed mindedness, the addict predictively continues downward. Of course, the same exact result is to be expected—only worse. Stuck in this quagmire of misery and despair, the addict's darkest void grows deeper and deeper.

However, after each destruction of the addict's

foundation, the addict's addiction starts failing, faltering. The addiction can only hide the addict's widening hole of darkness for mere moments at a time. These 'moments at a time' necessitate the addict's need to continue in the addiction at a quicker pace. This quickened pace leads to continuous dysfunction and inevitable, ongoing destruction, which causes an escalation of damage. It is therefore impossible to rebuild anything meaningful and lasting on such an imperfect foundation.

There is another choice the addict can finally make. Option #2 is to build on God's foundation. This is only possible in the addict's weakened state. This weakened state allows the spirit a voice of purity and enlightenment which the addict cannot ignore at this rare moment of vulnerability. This could be the spirit's final voice, a final chance to force the addict to admit to the "self" the real truth. The addict who choses Option #2 has now admitted and surrendered, which is giving up the addiction. Through the spirit's gasping resolve, the addict accepts and begins the climb back into God's sunshine.

On the climb up, regardless of how difficult it may be, the addict has now received God's love, warming and filling with lightness the void within. This is the only way out of addiction: GOD.

Soulo and the Spirit Whisperer

To "solo." A soloist is a person who is performing or tackling a task on their own. A soloist does not have anyone accompanying them for whatever task or activity they are doing. Again, this person is alone and accomplishing a goal. Usually, the solo act is done in commonly known activities such as music, flying, sports, etc.

Taking this standard definition of solo, and applying it in a singular, spiritual activity, is known as "soulo." The performing of "soulo" is based on a person who is unencumbered with day-to-day life and has the ability to stay in the moment while not letting worry or frustrations interfere with appreciating the blessings of daily living. "Souloing" is available to any human being who is ready to learn how to accomplish living on a higher, elevated plain of existence. This higher level of living is accessible to the ever-seeking spiritualist who has practiced being receptive to God's compass and has mastered, over time, being pure to the natural laws of the universe, the continuous cleansing of spiritual channels, and staying completely true to *self* through resolving all internal conflict.

In addition, to "soulo," one must have purged their old character and abandoned their old belief system that was based on negative principles. To achieve and attain this step, and rise to the next, elevated level among the many levels one can eventually reach, the individual, the souloist, must truly learn to listen to their voice's silence. Also, the new souloist engages in action based on listening to their God-given natural instincts. These steps allow the souloist to begin earning the complete trust of their spirit. The individual souloist has now begun to walk on God's one true path and is aware that this walk must be in a straighter line.

This next level of attainment can only be reached through constant evolution of the individual's soul and the commitment to daily spiritual exercise known as "pushups for the soul." These *pushups* are based on the individual continuing to be aware of God's presence in their life at all times, as well as constantly making the right instinctual choices. The habitual, instinctual choices, made without delay, are the principles behind spiritual exercises. The awareness and employment of these principles brings further spiritual insight and creates evolutionary growth for the soul.

Through the recognition of God's daily presence and blessings, an individual is put in touch with the natural laws of nature that guide their lives and their decisions. The souloist begins designing their life in a meaningful, fully respectful way of following God's plan for each human being. God's compass, instinctually designed "within self" points the individual to "true north." The true north of God's compass always points to the "beyonds of heaven" and keeps this spiritual, highly calibrated individual only on the one true path.

It is the mastery of understanding and awareness *without* effort. It is of "being in the entirety of each and every moment." It allows for the creation of perfect balance in one's life. This lifelong, lasting reward, when realized by the self, results in the seamless joining of one's life into God's harmonic plan of life.

This natural, instinctual bond of awareness enables the human being, when alone, to soulo. Soulo is the singular art of allowing the spirit and the individual to join together by exploring the here and now. The beginning souloist must practice stillness and allow the spirit within to emerge. The spirit has always been hiding in plain sight. To soulo brings the spirit together with the individual. To walk and be in *real truth*, the individual must rely on the trusting of self. Each individual souloist knows how to obtain internal peace by bringing about and achieving stillness of thought, which is considered to be the "idling of the conscience." At this point, when "idling," the conscience isn't consumed with any type of negativity or distraction. With the individual being still, the spirit is able to unite into souloist's presence and consciousness.

The souloist knows that, in order to begin real exploration and the *revealing of spirit*, it is essential to always be in the real truth and not deviate from the one true path. As the individual remains grounded in harmonic balance, the souloist is intensely aware of allowing the experience of thoughts and surroundings to be shared with the spirit and vice versa. Ultimately, souloing is strictly based on the souloist who is fully practiced and aware that they have obtained a rarified elevation of human consciousness. The tuned-in souloist on "higher ground" knows that the spirit permits this total oneness through truth, honesty, openness, and willingness. When the individual is souloing and allowing the spirit to be in charge, the souloist has learned to take a "back seat" during these journeys of uniting into one. In other words, the individual souloist has learned how to be fully engaged in this process by sitting back and letting the spirit be the guide and in charge. This allows the souloist to explore this new, uncharted state of being from a noble perspective.

This way of being present in the moment of *now* is considered to be a viewpoint from loftier heights than the spiritualist is accustomed to when alone and without the guidance of their spirit.

Once again, trust between the individual and spirit is not only necessary, it is the main component of having the freedom to soulo. The lapsing of real truth brought upon by the individual ignoring their instincts, side stepping or falling backward on the one true path leads to the spirit declining to be present and can eventually lead to spiritual hibernation. It is only through the individual's dedicated, disciplined work to continue on the one true path over a period of time that the spirit can once again be coaxed out of this hibernation.

The individual who has not been on the one true path as a result of not following God's instinctual compass must begin to listen to their natural instincts and begin to walk this one true path. Over time, through silent understanding, the individual will begin to intuitively feel the essence of God's hints and clues. With deep, meaningful progress, only then will the individual be in tune with the self to begin to learn and meet the requirements of how to be a "spirit whisperer."

As with the "horse whisperer" or "dog whisperer," the individual needs to develop trusting dialogue with the spirit within. This dialogue is in the language and action of real truth. The real truth dialogue is practiced by becoming more in tune with natural, truthful instincts that God has instilled in each human being. Actually performing these actions at all times, which are pure and beyond any individual's selfishness, results in the neglected spirit waking up. Keep in mind that the spirit whisperer is actually doing the listening to God's compass and acting on the individual's instinctive choices. Spirit whispering is spoken by the daily performing of positive actions that benefit and enrich the individual's human existence. It is through these thorough, daily actions that the self is actually "whispering" to the spirit. The individual following God's one true path in their daily thoughts and actions is actually the language being "whispered" to the spirit. The countless years of choosing the wrong choices and going against God's gifted instincts have corrupted and buried the self from the highest levels in which the spirit resides. To the resurrected individual, these new, daily actions walking down God's one true path wake the spirit within from its slumber.

It is important to keep the spirit awake initially by understanding that the individual's lifetime was spent making and doing the wrong moral activities, along with negative thoughts, causing the spirit within to withdraw from the individual's life. The individual's spirit does not trust at all, as the individual has broken the connection between self and God by walking the wrong path and following their own compass.

As the individual seeks a new, corrective course to live the life God guaranteed, the spirit makes its presence known . . . albeit rather slowly. As the individual shows to self their continuous progression on God's one true path, the spirit begins to intensify the individual's personal instincts, and in all reality the spirit is actually whispering back to the self. The more the individual listens to this spirit whispering, the more the individual whispers back to the spirit through these new, godly actions that are now becoming more instinctual. This is the bedrock of souloing, the spirit whispering between each internal entity that is creating wholeness of self. There is never that dark void within which in the past was filled temporarily by bad moments and choices. Eventually, through trust and more trust, this dark, gaping void within has been filled with the purest form of self . . . *oneness*. Spirit whispering is the mutual, ongoing trust and elevation of pure thought and direction between self and the spirit.

The souloing continues with the creation within of a deeper understanding of self. This spirit whispering enables the individual to walk God's one true path by instinctually following God's compass, leading to the divine richness of

201

life. Overtime, the spirit will take the lead, guiding the self. The spirit within knows how to productively wander the earth, along with the heavens, leading the individual to limitless "higher ground." The individual souloist knows to take a back seat for these experiences and travels. When souloing, the individual cannot falter or doubt this spiritual connection. Souloing cannot be interrupted by any type of questioning when traveling with the spirit to the highest of heights during any souloing session. If the souloist is mistrusting, wondering if the experience is imagined, or not able to achieve an absolute peaceful state of mind, it will cause the spirit to withdraw once again. The trust has been broken and the spirit whispering ends.

The individual must be vigilant in the creation and maintenance of balanced, peaceful thought. The individual must demonstrate purity of soul daily through truthful actions. Failure or any faltering on the one true path instantaneously sends the spirit back into hibernation.

Over a period of truthful encounters and exhibiting the purest truth, the spirit will emerge from within the self and actually allow the souloist to see, feel, and connect with the spirit. This lightened phase of spirit whispering makes the individual whole and as one with the self in totality for longer lengths of observable, unmeasured time. The final goal is to learn to be *one* at all times. Through this achievement, the spirit is of the "highest of light" and the individual, the souloist, is now soaring. The souloist is totally aware of the presence of their spirit, due to the spirit's illumination and the mutual trust established by spirit whispering. This is the purest form of souloing: to allow the spirit to be the guide as the individual sits back to take part in this majestic experience.

The souloist's journey, through timely, unexpected

practice, leads to the further exploration of self. The overall effect to self is a calming presence highlighted by a state of focused awareness while in the present moment. Regardless of the time or destination, the souloist is aware of the reality of the experience.

After souloing, the individual is back to the natural state of living their daily life, although the self is acutely aware of all the facts of the journey in which the individual has recently participated.

The progress and significance of the soulo can never be understated, regardless of whether an individual's awareness only consists of the spirit checking in with the souloist. It may only be during initial souloing that the presence of the spirit is felt. One of the main goals of the souloist is the total mastery of the individual self to participate as a spectator to the spirit's soaring. To the individual, there is never any doubt within self with regard to the overall experience. This holy experience always resonates within the self.

The individual, who is now totally aware of how to soulo through longer exercises of spirit, has developed an unquenchable desire to further the opportunity for more souloing. The individual now walks an even finer path with clarity. The individual follows their instinctual conscience within to continue to feed and nurture the spirit within self. The individual knows now that using real truth on God's one true path will begin another episode of this incredible, revealing journey. The souloist is on heightened alert to always be in the ready for instant unification from the spirit within. The individual staying exactly in the moment while walking the absolute path, along with practicing peace at all times, is suddenly, without any prompting, finding they are being summoned and the souloing has already begun.

Dana Axelrod

To soulo is a spiritual art form. Like any other modern-day soloist, the individual must be a master in their class or arena. Anyone who solos or *soulos* has taken the necessary steps to learn through daily practice how to improve their technique and chosen craft to perform for success under the spotlight of being alone. Enlightenment and exhilaration are only byproducts of this powerful experience, which is now imbedded within and never forgotten, only remembered.

God's Buffet

Everyone at one time in their lives has been to an all-you-can-eat buffet. Many diners continually go back to their favorite buffet over and over again. Others take the advice of people they respect and venture out and try a new venue. Those who do not go back to the buffet dining experience nevertheless remember the best dishes they enjoyed and the details of their particular buffet.

The reasons vary widely as to why buffets are so popular. The majority of diners enjoy the freedom to choose from a variety of their favorite dishes and that they can eat as much as they desire for one price. Simply pay one fee from your hard-earned cash and enjoy the entire meal. Of course, the only real drawback to any buffet is eating beyond your stomach's capacity, with the result being getting really, really stuffed.

The same conversations always take place after the buffet. Usually the conversation goes along the lines of, "I am so full," or "I should not have eaten so much. I need to go on a diet after that buffet," and finally, "I am so sick from eating so much."

However, there is another buffet where you never, ever get full. Regardless of how much is put on your plate. In fact, as you continually get served more and more, you actually get a bigger plate. The greatest pleasure at God's Buffet is that you never get full. This buffet is the one being served to you personally by God.

God's Buffet serves you your favorite dishes. These dishes are your blessings. The price you pay is not in monetary form like for a normal buffet where you spend your hard-earned cash. The price paid by the diner at God's Buffet is in the form of good deeds done daily toward yourself and others. In other words, your hard-earned cash is not used up like it is when you pay the bill at a normal buffet. At God's Buffet you receive your meals by giving toward yourself and others in a beautiful way. Talk about a rebate!

At your normal buffet we leave our home and travel to the restaurant. If we don't know the directions to the buffet, we plug in our GPS or use Google maps and follow the instructions. Following the GPS takes us to the buffet. We listen, follow the directions, make a left turn, a right turn, whatever type turn, and eventually, we arrive for our unlimited, all-you-can-eat buffet. After eating, we will most definitely say the same things: "I am so full, etc. etc."

At God's Buffet the directions are instilled inside us using God's Positioning System, otherwise known as our internal GPS. The directions we receive are calibrated by God's compass within. God's compass is always pointed toward showing each individual how to keep doing the right moral and spiritual actions. To get to dine at God's Buffet, we follow the easy-to-learn directions. These instructions are being told to us by our instincts and conscience. During this long road trip, we travel to God's Buffet on the one true path. When traveling on the one true path, we receive varying, healthy sustenance in the form of continuous appetizers and sampler plates. These free, delectable dishes are called daily blessings. These samplers or blessings keep us going on this beautiful highway of our life.

There are times in our life when we stop listening to God's compass inside ourselves and we get lost. We continue to ignore this beautiful voice inside telling us to follow God's compass and get back on the one true path. Many times we don't listen, we shut the internal GPS off, and then find ourselves so far from the path we once started out on. We are starving to death.

The problem is always our "self" saying, "I am not lost, I know the way." When we ignore God's compass and internal directions, we not only end up in the middle of nowhere, but everyone else we invited along also gets lost.

Think of it as if you were going to a new, normal buffet. It has been highly recommended, and you and your family have been waiting for this "special" day. The family is starved. You are driving and decide to take a shortcut and shut off the GPS or Google maps. Your whole family is in the car, telling you that you're lost and they're hungry, but you, as the driver, keep saying, "I know the way, I'm not lost." You keep driving downhill and then you end up on a dusty road in the middle of a desolate corn field. The entire family looks around and says to you, the driver, "Where are we? We're lost. We're hungry."

There is only one way to God's Buffet. When we take a different direction and stop following directions on our internal GPS, why wonder why we are so famished? The real truth is that we haven't listened to and followed God's compass. Can you imagine a ship captain at sea or a pilot of a commercial aircraft who decided they know the way and shut down or ignore the onboard compass and GPS? The ship at sea would crash onto the shore, smash onto the rocks, or get grounded in shallow water. The airline pilot would crash the airliner into a mountain or miss the runway and crash land the plane on the ground. When we as individuals stop listening and following God's compass and our instincts, the exact same thing happens. We get lost, grounded, smashed, and crashed.

Why is it so difficult to follow the purest and simplest of directions? The reason is that everyone who has stopped listening thinks they know a shortcut. We tell ourselves we don't need help getting to where we are going. Unfortunately for those who follow their own compass, they always insist they are going where they want. Never admitting to themself or anyone else that they are wrong, lost, and don't know the way. They refuse, regardless of how lost they are, to ask for help. The *real truth* is that these people know exactly where they are headed and where they will end up. Even though they are always saying how hungry they are, they are not willing to listen to instructions or follow directions to get fed the right way. They are starved and famished, refusing to go to God's Buffet, even though they can smell from far off the delectable aroma of the greatest meals waiting.

There is only one way to try to fill your plate with the deliciousness of God's blessings. Remember? The beauty of God's Buffet is that you never get full and you need—and receive—a bigger plate. The courses keep coming, day after day.

As we travel to God's Buffet on the one true path, we see, taste, and smell the oncoming meal for our entire lifetime. We stop to stretch our legs in life, enjoying the road. As travelers on God's one true path, we are fully aware of the appetizers and samplers we have snacked on and enjoyed as we continue to follow our internal GPS on the path to God's Buffet. The more we listen and follow the compass of God, the more we receive on our road trip, and our plates only get bigger.

Everyone who is following God's compass knows that at God's Buffet there are no terrible dishes to ignore, only our favorites. On the way to God's Buffet, we are only fed the most beautiful things in life. We never ask for more or something not on the menu. We have learned through listening and understanding that when we arrive at God's Buffet, the Chef of this establishment only serves each individual the dishes that will be enjoyed the most. Every dish is personally selected for each of the travelers. The dishes are made specifically to satisfy, excite, and make each participant imagine the wonders of life. We know at God's Buffet that there is only one purpose and that is to feed each of us beautiful courses throughout the entire meal.

In the normal buffet everyone picks and choses their personal, favorite dishes while ignoring others. At God's Buffet the Chef prepares and knows what each diner's favorite dishes are. The Chef knows what dishes each diner needs for nourishment. In addition, we are fully aware that the Chef has only our best interests at heart, and the dishes are prepared with what each individual needs in order to stay healthy and grow.

On the one true path, when we first start out, we are given sample appetizers. These appetizer blessings satisfy our hunger and make each individual, as we smack our lips, hungry for more. The individual on the one true path continues to receive delicate morsels, along with a dazzling array of "samplers." In fact, as the individual continues to listen to the directions from within and keeps receiving these delectable samplings, they are never hungry. The individual is no longer in a hurry to get to God's Buffet, as they are fed the entire time as they travel the one true path.

We are not full on the one true path at all; we are satisfied.

It is only when we stop following the directions and God's compass that we suddenly get hungry again. With the slightest veering off the one true path, the appetizers disappear, with the taste only lingering in our remembrance of them. The farther we go off the one true path, the more starved we suddenly get. If we have never been on the one true path, we are dying from malnutrition and anorexia due to *no real food*. We are always hungry for food that we know others have tasted on the way to God's Buffet.

At times on the way to God's Buffet, there are big billboards and advertisements claiming there is a better buffet. Sometimes, we are amazed how nice these rival billboards look and we decide to shut off our internal GPS. We follow others, take a very slight detour, and once again end up lost and starving. Other times, we head to those other buffets due to false advertising, how close they are, or how far away God's Buffet seems to be. The appetizers suddenly disappear, the sampler plate from God's Buffet is gone, and all that remains is the essence of that fine food that was awaiting our arrival.

Sometimes, the rival billboards and false advertisements are placed by the Chef of God's Buffet. These rival billboards placed by the Chef are to test your desire and see how starved you really are. Also, the Chef places these billboards and advertisements to see if the appetizers and sampler plates you have been eating on the one true path are enough to satisfy your appetite; He wants to see how much you really enjoyed them. For many, when the internal GPS is turned off and we eat at a different buffet, we leave and say, "I'm so full. I think I am going to be sick." Of course this does not happen at God's Buffet.

The more we listen and follow God's compass, the more appetizers and samplers we receive. Plates are groaning, overflowing under the weight of those tasty delicacies. Our plates runneth over. There is so much for each of us, with plenty to go around. We share, giving those appetizers to others. We are so grateful for those never-ending, all-day samplers and appetizers along the way to God's Buffet.

God is the Silence Between Peaceful Thoughts

We always hearing about "staying in the moment," the "here and now," and of course, "meaning and purpose." I was at a baseball game the other night, watching the game. I was "here" at the stadium right at that "moment." Looking around at all the cheering and booing fans drinking beer, snorkeling nachos, and hot dogs down their gullets, I said to myself, "All these thousands of people have a meaning and purpose right here, right now." The players on the field were also in the "here and now." Their purpose was to play their positions and win that particular game. Glancing at the manager, I saw that his "purpose" was to instruct and motivate his team to win. I thought, whoever loses, does that mean the team and/or the manager didn't stay in "the moment?" Didn't have "meaning and purpose?" The fans who are done eating and booing, is their meaning and purpose over?

I drive to the store, and I am in the moment. I have "purpose": my dog needs food. Is that making me in touch with my spiritual center? Am I Zen-like due to the fact that I recognize these things right now? It seems that whenever any individual is taking part in anything, good or bad, they are in "the moment." They are participating in the here and now. The criminal at the time of the crime has meaning and purpose.

Are all these aforementioned examples correct in my assumption of being in the here and now, in the moment, and having meaning and purpose? Basically, yes; emphatically, NO!

Really being in the moment, along with purpose and meaning, go way beyond those daily activities, regardless of whether those activities bring us joy or boredom. To really understand the principles of these words, it is important to open our viewpoint of everything we know, wipe the slate completely clean, and then dig deep inside ourselves.

Being in the moment with a clean personal slate is coming to terms with yourself as a human, spiritual being. To understand what the human spirit's real purpose is on this planet, you need to dig deep and ask, "What is this truly all about? What does it really mean to actively be placed on earth with the ceiling of God's Creation overhead?" To be alive and understand there is something far more involved in each of us, and it is more complex than going about living our daily lives.

To some, going to the job, paying bills, enjoying whatever it is anyone enjoys, is not enough. Every human spirit needs to question and begin to understand the answer. To find the answer to God's hints and clues, begin with your spirit simply looking up to the heavens, the universe, and start from that point with questions. Look up at night for only a few minutes and start the process of digging deep. Ask yourself a few simple questions about being in the "here and now" at this very moment. Don't bother trying to comprehend even one quadrillionth $(1/1,000,000,000,000,000^{th})$ of this universe's "meaning and purpose."

They enormity and perfect complexity of the universe is breathtaking and deserves the reverence given fine art works. This universe goes on and on, with or without any human being on earth. There is not a damn thing any human can do when it comes to the universe. We can fuck earth up and it will have no effect, no bearing whatsoever on the universe. The real truth is that the universe does not care, nor does earth have any control or even matter to this massive, mind-boggling creation of "art." What are we being shown? Why are we allowed to be a witness to this Creation? Look at it in an abstract way: does the universe exist, doing its colossal magic trick, without the human being aware of it? That is the only reason. That is the *hint*, the *clue*. The Creator wants us to be part of this spectacular, *live*, living Creation. Inter-active art between the artist and the spectator. This is where we begin to ponder and start understanding the *real truth*, God's truth of "purpose and meaning." This is when God wants us to be "in the moment," in the "here and now." This is the greatest game of virtual reality that exists; but it is not a game, it is *our* reality of "meaning and purpose."

To really understand ourselves, be ourselves, and follow God's purpose as spiritual beings, all we really need to do is think back and remember. Remember when you, the individual, lost consciousness while being totally awake. When you were sitting, thinking about *anything* for any amount of time, and suddenly, you said, "Damn . . . what was I thinking about? Where was I right then?" You were aware for a heartbeat, a minute, an hour, a day, that you had lost your awareness of thought and were . . . in *silent consciousness*. That is God! God is the Silence Between Peaceful Thoughts.

You go back for the briefest of time, trying to recall what you had been thinking. Maybe you remember and maybe you don't. That's irrelevant. What you should be trying to figure out is where you were during that "silence." That moment when time simply shifted. That is the real "here and now." That is the nano second when all shuts down and you, as a spiritual being, are simply in the perfect

213

moment of God's masterpiece within the "here and now." As a spiritual being, the more you are aware of this moment and prolong it, the more you will understand the real truth of why you are on earth.

Imagine if you could harness this moment of God's silence and could practice figuring out how to stay in that moment to grow and be more in touch with the Creator. The spirit is hungry for those moments of God's silence, and you have been practicing that moment for your entirety on earth. The key to this pureness of God's silence is the communication between God, the spirit, and the taking part in this universe. The self has let go of the restraining bonds of earthly thought and plugged the spirit into God's masterpiece.

That is called the *intellectual design of the consciousness of human thought*. To begin to reach this "spiritual time shift," start with your dreams and imagination. It doesn't matter the if or the what when it comes to your dreams. Fantasize, explore, feel, taste, be one inside any of your dreams. See the color of gold burning bright. Are there any limits on God's Creation, the universe? Of course not. The universe is limitless. It has a beginning (supposedly); however, no one has seen the end or figured out this entire art piece by the Master. To connect and be part of this master creation, where are the limits to the individual's dreams and imagination? Do we as individuals limit our dreams?

To understand the correlation between the self's imagination and God's silence, look at the anatomy of the brain. Look at all that humans know and how much is really understood about the exact functioning of this intellectually designed system. How much do the best and the brightest really know about the functioning of the brain? They have only scratched the surface of this intriguing, organic machine. They have no idea exactly how this complex machine instilled in the human being actually functions. The experts fail to understand the complexity of the brain.

Parallel this with what is known by the best and the brightest with regard to the universe. Aside from a multitude of theories by the best and the brightest on earth, no one has a clue or is an authority on this incredible spectacle. Perhaps there is a connection between the brain and the universe. This is where you begin to dig deep, understanding that now is the time to stimulate your imagination and start uniting your spirit, your soul, and the imagination of your mind. This is where you begin to create using balance, harmony, and the natural state within self. You are now creating the connection to receive, and you begin to feel God's "hints and clues." Through your personal creation of this harmonic pyramid within self, you begin to connect and be receptive to the energy of the Creation and now have become part of this master work. Much like meditation and the reaching of Nirvana, the balance of your receptive connection of energy will open your imagination up beyond the heavens to let your spirit soar. By allowing your intellectually designed mind to be fed and nourished, you are letting go of conscious thought to be one with God.

Everyone has been a passenger and put their hand out a car window to feel the wind, been on a motorcycle, or in a convertible going 60 mph. We felt this force *against* us. In the convertible or on a motorcycle, the sound of the wind rushing past our ears and on our faces made us conscious of the wind and our speed.

Use your imagination to connect and go with the wind while you are traveling as a passenger on earth at 67,000 mph! Do you realize how that rush sounds and feels to your ears and body while you are hurtling through the universe as an interactive participant in God's Creation?

That *is* the silence. That is being *one with*. That is being connected to God's universe. That silence is a deafening roar. Imagine where you have ended up after being a passenger on that ride, even if it is only for a nano second, or maybe, just maybe, perhaps it is at the speed of light. You figure it out. Imagination is the creative side of the brain that the Creator of All has instilled inside each of us.

Regardless of our circumstances on this planet, everyone has this universe inside their minds. Everyone. Unfortunately, billions of people on earth are tragically unaware and are victims of those circumstances. The spirit must be developed to the quiet understanding of being a guest participant in God's Creation. As a guest participant, you are being invited to witness the color of gold burning brightly and your 'self' being surrounded by that light. Where did you end up? Use your imagination. You will eventually know when you have arrived there. Where? *In the moment* with God, of course.

As human, spiritual beings sidestepping the tide pools of our lives, we are allowed and must give ourselves permission by using our imaginations to connect and soar. The real truth is that you can drop all of your manmade bullshit, good and bad, to unite yourself to be receptive to the silence of that moment in the "here and now" of the rushing wind. The stillness and absolute silence of that moment are deafening.

By exercising thought to the furthest level and beginning the wondering of what is deep down within self, take a look at the geniuses who have lived: Einstein, Da Vinci, Galileo—all succeeded where others did not. It was due to their elevation and personal understanding of their thought processes. That thought process is the intelligent design stimulated to the furthest outreaches of their imaginations. They touched the silence of God and were able to transform that energy by connecting and recharging their spirits into their own personal creations. Only through harmonious interaction between God's silence, the spirit, the soul, and the imagination can the human being create greatness which withstands time. This interacting connection is available to all who can wander into their imagination, who can hear and feel the silence. The ability to recognize and prolong the gaps of God's silence between thoughts is the most precious gift given to the individual spirit. There is no razor's edge, no limits or boundaries to the thoughts of imagination, as the imagination is endless, like the universe.

The goal is to harness this incredible silence and truly allow your spirit to continue to grow through touching and understanding the unspeakable God's silence and being *one*, in the moment of definitely the "here and now." That *is* the "meaning and purpose" of all of our lives. To be able to shed all the layers off our own spirit and let the purity of our spirit show God's brightness through us. The "hints and clues" are revealed, along with the answers, through those geniuses who have connected.

Michelangelo's statue of David is considered by many to be the most "lifelike" statue of man ever created. Michelangelo, when asked how he was able to create such a lifelike, godly image of man, replied, "The statue was in the rock, I simply chipped it out."

There are all of our answers. The godly spirit is inside each of us, and as human beings, we must chip away at the years and all the endless layers of bullshit each of us has wrapped around our souls. However, with so little time on earth to "get it right," chipping is not an option. The only real answer to truly free the spirit is to use a sledgehammer on yourself. Smash the hardened rock encasing your mind and spirit to begin to really dream. Michelangelo again answers another "hint and clue" for all of us in the painting called the "Creation of Adam." Regardless of the religious connotation focus on the manmade art, the painting simply shows God touching His finger to the finger of Adam. Is it by chance that God is pictured inside the human brain? What more do any of us need? Let God touch you through the Creation. The silence.

When you hear that silence, then your spirit knows. That is the passion, the inspiration your spirit thirsts for to unite with human nature and guide you on earth. There are no more doubts or fears when you have been touched to take an active part in the Creator's Creation. Regardless of whether you re-encase your mind and spirit in concrete again. It is too late, as you now know. Deep down you really, really know. Those who are elevated and receptive as a result of their sledgehammering will dream bigger and always imagine further. By understanding and emerging through the silence, the spirit's future is in the self's hands.

The self who embraces those silent tours of distant art walk with "purpose and meaning." The self is *believing* who it is, not *doubting*, has *faith* in self, *knows* the answer, and is a human who is *being*. The self has the perfect balance of the natural law of the universe and is truly *shining*.

ABOUT THE AUTHOR

Dana started his road into addiction by experimenting with drugs and alcohol at the early age of 13. Dana states, "I became more involved with drugs and alcohol to 'fit in' with all the other loners and misfits". By the age of 21, Dana was on a life long, descent as he spiraled downward into the bleak existence of alcohol and drug addiction.

Alcohol, drugs, and more drugs was the only priority in Dana's everyday life. Regardless of Dana's escalating consumption of alcohol and illicit drugs, Dana was able to work with Hollywood's biggest stars on countless films, tv shows, commercials, and music videos. Dana continued to recklessly stumble his way to the top of the film business joining the Director's Guild of America. Eventually, Dana's professional and personal life came shattering down in a haze of OD's, arrests, and family dysfunction.

Checking himself into 'rehab' Dana decided to understand thoroughly the exact nature of his and other's addictions along with the reasons and behaviors behind all addictions. After 'rehab' Dana retired from the Director's Guild of America after 25 years and says, "My addiction robbed me of my dreams, my goals, and the elevation of professional success. On the set, my mind was always thinking of the next 'dose' or counting the hours until I could get drunk." This was the beginning of Dana's quest to understand all addictions by enrolling in college to become a certified Drug and Alcohol counselor.

Dana has gone on to be a positive influence to others and has achieved global recognition while winning numerous awards in the Drug and Alcohol field. In 2017 and again in 2021 Dana won the prestigious 'Residential Counselor of the Year' awarded by the California State Assembly. In addition, Dana has won the 'Healer of the Year' award along with being recognized and rewarded by the Brother's of Saint John of God resulting in a 10 day trip to Granada, Spain to 'Follow in the Footsteps of St John of God' the patron Saint of Hospitality.

Today, Dana continues to motivate and inspire others to 'pursue their dreams'. Dana currently lectures, counsels individuals, families, and groups on addiction, spirituality, and positive change from his locale in San Diego.

THANKS AND REMEMBRANCES

MY THANKS TO: Jordan Weiner, Joshua Hanson, Will Harper, Anita and the Tolbert family, Alex and the entire Atalla family, Ayham and Khatam Dahi, the Scibella clan, the Axelrod tribe, Pastor Tom Mercer and family, Dr. Craig Mueller, Teressa Johnston, Edward and Shirley Oleschak, Ross Judd, Chris Burton, Ms. Marinor Ifurung, Kenny Bryant, Terry Hurst, Thomas Salas, Shannon Davis, Santiago Lopez, Tony Perez III and family, Brandi Devlin, Debbie Archuletta, Lary Croutch, Micah Bass, Janice DiGrande, Teresa and Curtis Lange, Larry Mangiapane, Gary Worland, Ms. Charlotte, Ms. Anna, Ms. Cynthia, Ms. Jackie Sharitts, Billy, Ms. Yvette, Sunny Hatten, Kathleen Miller, Sonya Hernandez, Samantha Davis, Toby Slater, H.B. Barnum, Eothen Alapatt, Kristoff Indeherberge, Dr. May and Lhema Mayouda, Roxy and Marc at Fred Brown Recovery, Tom Brady (The GOAT), and my most trusted, silent associate, Emmitt.

SPECIAL THANKS TO: my editor, Ms. Jenny Margotta

TO THE "PATRIOTS" WHO TOOK PART IN THEIR OWN REVOLUTION AND JOINED ME IN GOD'S ARMY: Derek Fowler, Mia Bryant, Cassie Bates, Marco DeLarosa, Enrique and Pauline Vega, Dixie Bolen, Brandon Gwynn, Ivan Urtuastegui, and of course, Tommy Black, *and all the other addicts who opened their minds and their hearts, and trusted me.*

Dana Axelrod

RIP: Scott Axelrod, Kinda Atalla, Rocky Atalla, Frank Scibella, Kenny Ostin, Gary Flasher, Neil Michael, Ryan Dorff, Tony Scibella, James Tolbert, David Axelrod, Radwa and Rezkalla Atalla, Oscar Strange, Joan Scibella, Bob Burner, Dave Hanson, Keith Dillon, Greg Barnes, Whitney Houston, and Gus.